Dosage Calculations for Nurses

Visit the *Dosage Calculations for Nurses* Companion
Website at **www.pearsoned.co.uk/olsen** to find valuable
student learning material including:

+ Self-assessment questions to help test your learning
+ Links to relevant sites on the web
+ Additional case studies
+ A guide to student success

Dosage Calculations for Nurses

June L. Olsen MS, RN
Professor of Nursing (Emeritus)
College of Staten Island, Staten Island, NY

Anthony Patrick Giangrasso PhD
Professor of Mathematics
LaGuardia Community College, Long Island City, NY

Dolores M. Shrimpton MA, RN
Professor of Nursing
Chairperson, Department of Nursing
Kingsborough Community College, Brooklyn, NY

Patricia M. Dillon MA, RN
Professor of Nursing
Deputy Chairperson, Department of Natural and Applied Science
LaGuardia Community College, Long Island City, NY

Sheila Cunningham RN MSc, PGDipEd FHEA
Principal Lecturer
School of Health and Social Sciences
Middlesex University, London, United Kingdom

Harlow, England • London • New York • Boston • San Francisco • Toronto
Sydney • Tokyo • Singapore • Hong Kong • Seoul • Taipei • New Delhi
Cape Town • Madrid • Mexico City • Amsterdam • Munich • Paris • Milan

Pearson Education Limited
Edinburgh Gate
Harlow
Essex CM20 2JE
England

and Associated Companies throughout the world

Visit us on the World Wide Web at:
www.pearsoned.co.uk

First published 2010

ISBN: 978-0-13-206884-0

British Library Cataloguing-in-Publication Data
A catalogue record for this book is available from the British Library

Library of Congress Cataloging-in-Publication Data
Dosage calculations for nurses / June L. Olsen . . . [et al.].
    p. ; cm.
  Includes bibliographical references and index.
  ISBN 978-0-13-206884-0 (pbk.)
  1. Pharmaceutical arithmetic.   2. Nursing–Mathematics.   I. Olsen, June Looby.
  [DNLM: 1. Pharmaceutical Preparations–administration & dosage–
Nurses' Instruction.   2. Pharmaceutical Preparations–administration &
dosage–Problems and Exercises. 3. Mathematics–Nurses' Instruction.
4. Mathematics–Problems and Exercises.   QV 18.2 D722 2010]
  RS57.D6695 2010
  615'.1401513–dc22

                                                                    2009025898

10 9 8 7 6 5 4 3 2 1
13 12 11 10 09

Typeset in 9.5/12pt Din Regular by 35
Printed in Great Britain by Henry Ling Ltd, at the Dorset Press, Dorchester, Dorset

The publisher's policy is to use paper manufactured from sustainable forests.

For my three girls, with love: Larissa, Michelle, and Taylor.
June Looby Olsen

*To Carlos Arevalo, James Kwee, and George Rivara: good tennis
buddies, great physicians, and even better human beings.*
Anthony Giangrasso

*To my son, Shawn, daughter-in-law, Kim, granddaughters,
Brooke Elizabeth and Paige Dolores, and our newest addition Jack Paul
for all the love and happiness they have brought into my life.*
Dolores M. Shrimpton

*To my husband, Patrick, and daughters Leigh Ann and Katie,
for their enduring patience and loving support, and to my colleague,
Sheila Acheson, for inspiration.*
Patricia M. Dillon

*Andrew, Kathy, Lizzie and Mark – thanks for your support,
encouragement and often interesting suggestions.*
Sheila Cunningham

Contents

Unit 2
Oral and parenteral medications

Supporting resources

Visit **www.pearsoned.co.uk/olsen** to find valuable online resources

Companion Website for students

+ Self-assessment questions to help test your learning
+ Links to relevant sites on the web
+ Additional case studies
+ A guide to student success

Also: The Companion Website provides the following features:

+ Search tool to help locate specific items of content
+ E-mail results and profile tools to send results of quizzes to instructors
+ Online help and support to assist with website usage and troubleshooting

For more information please contact your local Pearson Education sales representative or visit **www.pearsoned.co.uk/olsen**

About the authors

JUNE LOOBY OLSEN began her nursing career in Burlington, Vermont, at Bishop De Goesbriand Memorial Hospital, where she graduated from its Nursing Programme. She obtained her BS and MS degrees in nursing from St. John's University, New York. She was a staff nurse, nurse supervisor, and became Head Nurse at the Veterans Administration Hospital in Brooklyn, New York.

Her teaching career began at Staten Island Community College, and she retired as Full Professor Emeritus from the College of Staten Island of the City University of New York. In addition to this textbook, Professor Olsen has written, *Fundamentals of Nursing Review* and *Dosage Calculation* both published by Springhouse. She was a recipient of the Mu Epsilon Leadership in Nursing award.

ANTHONY GIANGRASSO was born and raised in Maspeth, NY. He attended Rice High School on a scholarship, and in his senior year was named in a citywide contest by the *New York Journal-American* newspaper as New York City's most outstanding high school scholar-athlete. He was also awarded a full-tuition scholarship to Iona College, from which he obtained a BA in mathematics, magna cum laude, with a ranking of sixth in his graduating class.

Anthony began his teaching career as a fifth-grade teacher in Manhattan as a member of the Christian Brothers of Ireland, and taught high school mathematics and physics in Harlem and Newark, NJ. He possesses an MS and PhD from New York University, and has taught at all levels from elementary school to graduate school. He is currently teaching at Adelphi University and LaGuardia Community College, where he was chairman of the mathematics department. He has authored seven college textbooks.

Anthony's community service has included membership on the Boards of Directors of the Polish-American Museum Foundation, Catholic Adoptive Parents Association, and Family Focus Adoptive Services. He was the president of the Italian-American Faculty Association of the City University of New York, and the founding Chairman of the Board of the Italian-American Legal Defense and Higher Education Fund, Inc. He and his wife, Susan, are proud parents of three children Anthony, Michael, and Jennifer. He enjoys tennis, and in 2002 was ranked number one for his age group in the Eastern Section by the United States Tennis Association.

DOLORES M. SHRIMPTON is a professor and chairperson of the Department of Nursing at Kingsborough Community College of the City University of New York. She has been a nurse for more than 35 years and received a diploma in nursing from the Kings County Hospital Center School of Nursing. She obtained a BS degree from C. W. Post College and an MA degree in nursing administration from New York University. She also has a post-Master's certificate in nursing education from Adelphi University. She is a member of the Upsilon and Mu Upsilon Chapters of Sigma Theta Tau.

Dolores is the immediate past president of the New York State Associate Degree Nursing Council, where she also served as the vice president and member of its board of directors. She is the co-chair of the CUNY Nursing Discipline Council and an active member of the Nurses Association of the Counties of Long Island (NACLI), D 14 of the New York State Nurses Association. She serves on a number of advisory boards of LPN, associate degree, and baccalaureate degree nursing programs. She is also the project codirector of the New York State Coalition for Nursing Educational Mobility (NYSCNEM).

Dolores has received many awards for her achievements in nursing. She is a recipient of the Presidential Award in Nursing Leadership from NACLI, the Mu Upsilon award for Excellence in Nursing Education, and the 2006 Mu Upsilon award for Excellence in Nursing Leadership. Dolores has taught a wide variety of courses in practical nursing, diploma, and associate degree nursing programmes. Her area of clinical practice is maternity, with a focus on labour and delivery.

Dolores lives in Brooklyn, NY, and especially enjoys spending time with her grandchildren, Brooke Elizabeth, Paige Dolores, and Jack Paul, and their parents, Kim and Shawn.

PATRICIA M. DILLON As far back as she can remember, Pat always loved mathematics and science, and after getting a Regents Scholarship in Nursing, she decided that fate wanted her to choose that career. She obtained her BS in Nursing from Lehman College and MA from New York University.

Paediatric surgery became Pat's specialty at New York University Medical Center, where she also worked in neurosurgery, and finally in maternity. Her 22 years of experience in education began at Molloy College, followed by 4 years at Interfaith School of Nursing in Brooklyn, and to her longest position of 16 years in the Nursing Program at LaGuardia Community College. While there, she moved through the ranks from Assistant Professor of Nursing to her present position as Professor and Natural Applied Sciences Deputy Chair of Nursing. During her earlier years, she created a medical dosages video for Dimensional Analysis, which the nursing students found to be a very valuable learning supplement.

Pat has always been deeply involved in professional nursing organisations. Her numerous positions have included vice chairperson of the Parent-Child Health Nursing Clinical Practice Unit of New York State Nurses Association (NYSNA), as well as a 4–year term as chair of the same NYSNA PCHN-CPU Committee. She was later appointed chair of NYSNA's Council on Nursing Practice and an auxiliary member of the NY State Board of Nursing. Her awards include the Ruth W. Harper Distinguished Service Award for Commitment to Professional Excellence and Leadership from the Nurses Association of the Counties of Long Island (NACLI), NYSNA Local District 14, as well as the NYSNA 2004 Student's Choice Award. In 2006, she was inducted into the New York State Nurses Association Leadership Institute.

SHEILA CUNNINGHAM trained as a nurse at the Royal Free Hospital School of Nursing in London and had a varied clinical nursing career specialising in cancer nursing following further education at the Royal Marsden Hospitals in London and Surrey. In the early 1990s Sheila undertook the Postgraduate Certificate in Education at the Royal College of Nursing (Institute for Advanced Nursing Education) and has been working in education ever since, initially at the North London College of Health Studies, and continuing to do so when this became part of Middlesex University. Sheila was awarded a Teaching Fellowship in 2004 for excellence in teaching which is something she strives to pursue. She is also a fellow of the Higher Education Academy.

Preface

In a growing range of healthcare settings, nursing and allied health professionals are assuming increasing responsibilities for every aspect of medication administration. One important step in assuming this responsibility is learning to calculate drug dosages accurately and safely. Dosage calculation is not just about mathematical skills; it is grounded in confidence and understanding of the **professional context** of drug administration. Many nurses lack confidence which the safety of a simply explained book with workable examples can give them. The application to practice is critical, however more important is the application to all areas of life in which calculations are performed, and then from the familiar transfer those skills to more unfamiliar situations. Safety is paramount, both of the nurse and of the clients thus a safe practice area with step by step instructions is provided within this text.

Dosage Calculations for Nurses is a combined text and workbook of dosage calculations designed for the student. Its consistent focus on safety, accuracy, and professionalism make it a valuable part of a dosage calculation course for nursing or allied health programmes. It is also highly effective for independent study and may be used as a refresher to dosage calculation skills or as a professional reference.

Dosage Calculations for Nurses is arranged into three basic learning units:

Unit 1: Basic calculation skills and introduction to medication administration
Chapters 1 and 2 review basic mathematics skills and introduce the essentials of drug administration. Chapter 3 introduces fractions manipulations using a friendly, common sense approach.

Chapter 4 presents the metric system of measurement that nurses and other allied health professionals must understand to interpret medication prescriptions and calculate dosages.

Unit 2: Oral and parenteral medications
Chapters 5, 6, 7, and 8 prepare students to calculate oral and parenteral dosages and introduce them to the essential equipment needed for administration and preparation of solutions.

Unit 3: Infusions and paediatric dosages
This important final unit provides a solid foundation for calculating intravenous and enteral flow rates, and duration of infusions (Chapters 9 and 10). Paediatric dosages and daily fluid maintenance needs are discussed in Chapter 11.

Topics introduced and developed in *Dosage Calculations for Nurses* include:

+ basic arithmetic skills;
+ systems of measurement;
+ dosage calculations for all common forms of drug preparations;
+ IV and specialised calculations.

In addition to these topics, this edition includes substantially more information about safety in medication administration and follows the NMC Standards for Medicines Management, Medicines and Healthcare Products Regulatory Agency (MHRA) Label Guidance, and Department of Health Medication Safety guidance and recommendations. Readers will learn how to interpret actual drug labels, package inserts and patient information leaflets, and various forms of medication prescriptions, as well as how to select the appropriate equipment to administer the prescribed dose.

Benefits of using *Dosage Calculations for Nurses*

+ Constant skill reinforcement through frequent practice opportunities.
+ More than 1000 problems for students to solve.
+ Actual drug labels, syringes, drug package inserts.
+ Practice reading prescriptions and generalised medication administration records (MARs) throughout the text.
+ Work space on every page for problem solving.
+ Solutions to problems are found in Appendix A.

Acknowledgements

The publisher would especially like to thank Carol Lincoln for her contribution to the development of Chapter 2 of this textbook.

We would also like to thank the reviewers for their comments:

Amy Dopson, University of Surrey
Dr Margaret Edwards King's College London
Janet Holt, Leeds University

We are grateful to the following for permission to reproduce copyright material:

Figures
Figures 2.2, 2.10, 2.13, Epivir label on page 113, Retrovir label on page 113, Avandia label on page 116 and figures 8.7b and 11.8 from GlaxoSmithKline, reproduced with permission of GlaxoSmithKline; Figures 2.12, 2.17, Norvir label on page 115 and figure 5.6 from Abbott Laboratories Ltd, reproduced with permission; Figures 2.14, 8.4 and 9.13c from Merck Sharp & Dohme Ltd, reproduced with permission; Figure 2.20 from Actavis UK Ltd, reproduced with permission; Figure 2.15 reproduced with permission, Merck Sharp & Dohme Ltd; Figure 4.1 from Napp Pharmaceuticals Limited, reprinted with the permission of Napp Pharmaceuticals Limited; Figure 4.2, Diovan and Sandostatin labels on page 115 and Figure 5.2 from Novartis Pharmaceuticals Ltd, reproduced with permission of Novartis; Figure 5.3, Istin label on page 115, Figures 5.10, 8.7d, 9.13b and 10.4 reprinted with permission, courtesy of Pfizer Limited; Figures 5.4 and C.5 used with permission from Lundbeck Ltd UK; Cymbalta® label on page 112, Prozac® label on page 112 and figures 5.1 and 6.25a from Eli Lilly & Company, © Copyright Eli Lilly and Company. All rights reserved. Used with permission. ® CYMBALTA, PROZAC and HUMALOG are registered trademarks of Eli Lilly and Company; Zyprexa label on page 113, Figures 6.13, 6.17, 6.21, 7.7b and 7.7c © Eli Lilly & Company Ltd; Losec label on page 114 courtesy of AstraZeneca; Lanoxin label on page 114 and Figures 7.8 and 8.3 from Aspen Pharmacare, reproduced with permission from Aspen; Figure 6.23 diagram reprinted with kind permission from sanofi-aventis; Actrapid and Insulatard labels on page 142 used with permission from Novo Nordisk; Figure 7.7a reproduced with permission of Meda Pharmaceuticals Ltd; Figure 8.5 from Drug administration general principles in *The Royal Marsden Hospital Manual of Clinical Nursing Procedures* edited by Doughty, L. and Lister, S., 6th ed., Wiley-Blackwell (Lister, S. 2004), reproduced with permission; Figure 9.3 courtesy of Abbott Nutritional Services; Figures 9.4b, 9.5a, 9.5b, 9.5c, 9.5d, 9.9 and 9.10 courtesy of Baxter Healthcare Ltd; Figures 9.4c and 9.8b from Al Dodge/Al Dodge Photography; Figures 9.8a, 9.11, 10.2a and 10.2b images provided courtesy of Baxter Healthcare Corporation, reproduced with permission. Baxter Healthcare cannot assume any liability for the correct use of these labels in certain jurisdictions; Figure 11.3 reproduced with permission of Amdipharm Plc; Figure 11.5 Nomogram modified from data of E. Boyd by C. D. West, This article was published in

Nelson Textbook of Pediatrics, 16th ed., Behrman, R.E., Kliegman, R. M. and Jenson, H. B., Copyright Elsevier 2000.

Tables
Table 11.1 from *APA Consensus Guidelines on Perioperative Fluid Management in Children*, v.1.1, accessed online version March 2008, APAGBI (2007), reproduced with permission.

Text
Case Study 1.1 from *Building a Safer NHS for Patients: Improving Medication Safety – A Report by the Chief Pharmaceutical Officer*, Crown (2003), Crown copyright, Crown Copyright material is reproduced with the permission of the Controller of HMSO and the Queen's Printer for Scotland.

In some instances we have been unable to trace the owners of copyright material, and we would appreciate any information that would enable us to do so.

Unit 1

Basic calculation skills and introduction to medication administration

Chapter 1

Review of arithmetic skills for medical dosage calculations

Learning outcomes

After completing this chapter, you will be able to

1. Revise basic mathematical functions.
2. Convert fractions to decimal numbers and decimal numbers to fractions.
3. Round off decimal numbers to a desired number of places.
4. Multiply and divide decimal numbers.
5. Multiply and divide fractions.
6. Simplify complex fractions.
7. Write percentages as fractions or decimal numbers.

Mathematics and calculations are used daily, from calculating the correct change following shopping purchases to altering volumes in recipes to ensure we have enough food to feed people or planning a journey to arrive on time. Many of us use mathematics or calculations daily and do not realise we are doing it.

Mathematics, and particularly medical dosage calculations, are seen as complicated and difficult because they often involve fractions, decimal numbers and percentages. Many of us have developed fears and negative thoughts or feelings when hearing the word 'mathematics'. However, this fear can be overcome once you realise the range of everyday activities in which you perform mathematics or calculations and, with practice, you will become confident and competent in performing calculations following some basic rules. For those who wish to refresh their understanding of the basic mathematical concepts this chapter will be a useful reminder; for others with more confidence they may wish to skim through it taking what they wish from it along the way.

Diagnostic test of arithmetic

Before the chapter begins try to work out the following to establish your comfort with numbers:

1. Write 0.375 as a fraction. _____

2. Round off 6.492 to the nearest tenth. _____

3. $0.038 \times 100 =$ _____

4. Write $2\frac{1}{2}\%$ as a decimal number. _____

5. Write $2\frac{4}{7}$ as an improper fraction. _____

Check your answers and compare them with those at the end of the book in Appendix A. If you feel weak in any of these then work though this chapter at your own pace.

Fundamental skills for calculations

Numeracy is an important skill, not only for drug calculations but also for interpreting and evaluating data from patients, research, literature and generally managing life (finances, etc.). Hutton (2005) states that for nurses in particular there are four basic elements in calculation proficiency: common sense and estimation, the ability to perform mental arithmetic, use of a calculator (to check answers) and understanding the right formula to use. It is important to have an idea of what a sensible answer should be but also the ability to check, double check and, if necessary, ask for help. Standard 8 of the Standards for Medicines Management (NMC, 2007: 24) emphasises that some drug administrations can require complex calculations to ensure that the correct volume or quantity of medication is administered. Thus practice and confidence are important. Furthermore, it is good practice for a second practitioner (a registered professional) to check the calculation independently in order to minimise the risk of error. The use of calculators to determine the volume or quantity of medication, however, should not act as a substitute for mathematical knowledge and skill.

The fundamental skills required for numeracy or mathematical ability are recognition of mathematical symbols, how to use them and in what order. Consider the following problem:

$$4 + 2 \times 3 = ?$$

If we calculate $4 + 2$ first, then $\times 3$ we get:

$$4 + 2 = 6$$
$$6 \times 3 = \mathbf{18}$$

If we calculate 2×3 first, then $+ 4$ we get:

$$2 \times 3 = 6$$
$$6 + 4 = \mathbf{10}$$

Which one is correct? They are obviously two very different answers and, if this were a situation in a shop or restaurant, we would question our payment (£18 or £10). This may have other implications, for instance when calculating drug doses based on body weight; this would be almost double the dose difference and may be potentially harmful.

From school level mathematics you may remember the agreed order of actions as: addition, subtraction, division, etc. (also known as mathematical operations or functions). There is a useful acronym BODMAS to prompt us with this in cases of panic at where to start. BODMAS stands for the types of operations:

Brackets **O**ther **D**ivision and **M**ultiplication **A**ddition and **S**ubtraction

All these terms are fairly obvious apart from 'Other' which can be said to refer to operators such as powers or roots (e.g. 3^2 or 4^3 or $\sqrt{91}$).

Example 1.1

Work out the following:

$$4 + \frac{70}{10} \times (1 + 2)^2 - 1 = ?$$

This looks scary, but focus on the BODMAS steps and it is easy to work out:

Brackets first, thus:	$4 + \frac{70}{10} \times (3)^2 - 1$
Other next, thus:	$4 + \frac{70}{10} \times 9 - 1$
Division next, thus:	$4 + 7 \times 9 - 1$
Multiplication next, thus:	$4 + 63 - 1$
Addition then so:	$67 - 1$
Subtraction finally:	$\underline{66}$ is the answer

Note that Multiplication and Division have the same importance and so do Addition and Subtraction; so always answer the problem from LEFT to RIGHT so you know which to do first (multiplication or division, addition or subtraction).

Example 1.2

In the classroom you are discussing normal lung volumes. You have been asked to use a formula (based on Kendrick and Smith, 1992) to predict your Forced Vital Capacity (FVC), a respiratory volume based on maximum breath in and maximum breath out and measured in litres. Your height is 1.65 metres and you are a 24 year old female. The formula is:

$$\text{FVC (L)} = (4.43 \times \text{Height}) - (0.026 \times \text{Age}) - 2.89$$

This looks scary, but approach it logically; first insert the height and age where the words are, this should look like this:

$$\text{FVC} = (4.43 \times 1.65) - (0.026 \times 24) - 2.89$$

Using BODMAS steps the remainder should look like this:

Brackets first, thus:	$7.30 - 0.624 - 2.89$
Other next:	(none)
Division:	(none)

Multiplication next:	(none)
Addition:	(none)
Subtraction:	<u>3.78</u> L is the answer

Stop and think

Nurses and other healthcare professionals use mathematical calculations all the time and use the BODMAS rule quite naturally. Think about the calculation for Body Mass Index which is used frequently in clinical areas: Weight/(Height^2) = m^2 (weight in kgs divided by height in metres squared). Using the BODMAS rules, the height is identified and squared (do this first as it is in brackets), then divided into the weight giving a reading in metres squared (m^2).

Explaining decimals and fractions

Understanding of decimal numbers has been identified as a foundation for correct medicine or drug calculations, and practice with use of decimal numbers improves this ability (Pierce *et al.* 2008). You may be familiar with or even doing calculations of body mass index (see Stop and Think) or may be calculating a person's hip to waist ratio as a risk for heart disease (central obesity) yet did not realise you were using fractions to do this. This section will practise with fractions and how they are then incorporated into other calculations of clinical relevance.

A number can be written in different forms: a decimal, a fraction or a whole number. A whole number is straightforward: 1, 2, 3, 10, 99, etc. In general, a decimal and a fraction indicate a part of a whole number. When referring to a third of something we understand this is one part of something that has been divided into three, also written as: $^1/_3$. In their simplest form, fractions refer to parts of a 'whole'. Look at the following examples to refresh your memory.

Example 1.3

This long box has been divided into 8 equal parts. What fraction of the long box is shaded?

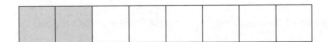

The long box has been divided into 8. So each small piece is $\frac{1}{8}$ of the whole long box. There are 2 parts shaded. So 2 of the $\frac{1}{8}$s are shaded. This means the fraction will have 2 on the top.

So the fraction of the long box that is shaded is $\frac{2}{8}$.

Example 1.4

If the long box had been cut into 4 pieces and one piece shaded then it would look like this.

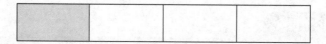

The fraction for this is $\frac{1}{4}$. We can compare the two fractions by putting them next to each other like this.

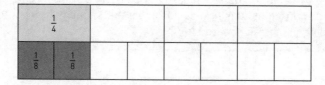

You can see that the amount shaded is the same in each strip. This means that the fractions are the same.

So $\frac{2}{8}$ is the same value as $\frac{1}{4}$. One can also write this as $\frac{2}{8} = \frac{1}{4}$.

A decimal is a number in the number system we are familiar with which has the base of 10 – this may have emerged to understand numbers and amounts because counting on ten fingers is easier! A decimal number is a fraction with a division of 10, 100, 1000, and so on. However, it is often not written as a fraction and has a particular notation involving a decimal point. Each decimal number has three parts: the whole number part, the decimal point and the fraction part. Consider the number 345. The construction of the number 345 actually means:

$$3 \text{ of } 100\text{s} + 4 \text{ of } 10\text{s} + 5 \text{ of ones}$$

Look at this number: 0.65.

Units(ones)	Decimal point	Tenths/10th	Hundredths/100th
0	.	6	5

The construction of this decimal part of a decimal number means

$$\frac{6}{10} + \frac{5}{100}$$

An everyday example of where decimal places can be seen in practice is with money: 100 pence equals one pound (£) or alternatively written 100p = £1.00. You may be shopping and have to decide which is the best bargain: get three for the price of two (or 40% off). Table 1.1 shows the names of the decimal positions.

Table 1.1 Names of decimal positions

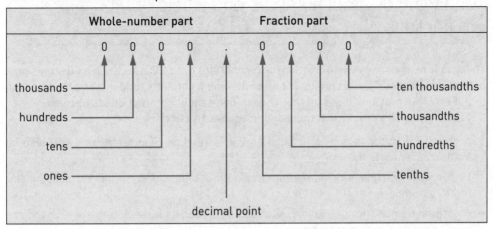

A fraction is composed of 2 parts: the **Numerator** – *the number on the top of the frac-tion* – and the **Denominator** – *the number on the bottom*. 'Reading' a decimal number will help you write it as a fraction (Table 1.2).

Table 1.2 Relating decimal numbers to fractions

Decimal number	⟶	Read	⟶	Fraction
4.1	⟶	four and one tenth	⟶	$4\frac{1}{10}$
0.3	⟶	three tenths	⟶	$\frac{3}{10}$
6.07	⟶	six and seven hundredths	⟶	$6\frac{7}{100}$
0.231	⟶	two hundred and thirty-one thousandths	⟶	$\frac{231}{1000}$
0.0025	⟶	twenty-five ten thousandths	⟶	$\frac{25}{10\,000}$

Stop and think

Which is larger 0.75 or 7.5?   (Answer 7.5 because 0.75 is smaller than 1)

Which is smaller 0.625 or 0.0625?   (Answer 0.0625 because the position of the 6 is in the hundreth place not the tenth place after the decimal point)

If these were medications then you would need to know the value of these numbers and the role of the decimal point in order to give the correct amount.

Changing decimal numbers and whole numbers to fractions

There may be instances when fractions are important in healthcare, such as decreasing a patient's dietary sodium intake by 1/3 or evaluating a patient's fluid intake and reporting that it is $^1/_2$ the previous day's intake. Thus understanding of fractions is necessary.

Fractions can be **proper fractions** and **improper fractions**:

+ A decimal number less than 1, such as 0.9, is read as nine tenths and can also be written as a *proper fraction* $\frac{9}{10}$.

    In a *proper fraction*, the *numerator* (top number) is *smaller* than its *denominator* (bottom number).

+ A decimal number greater than 1, such as 3.5, is read as three and five tenths and can also be written as the mixed number $3\frac{5}{10}$ or $3\frac{1}{2}$. A **mixed number** combines a whole number and a proper fraction. The mixed number $3\frac{1}{2}$ can be changed to a an *improper fraction* as follows:

$$3\frac{1}{2} = \frac{3 \times 2 + 1}{2} = \frac{7}{2}$$

    In an *improper fraction* the *numerator* (top number) is *larger* than the *denominator* (bottom number).

+ Any number can be written as a fraction by writing it over 1. For example, 9 can be written as the *improper fraction* $\frac{9}{1}$.

Example 1.5

Write 2.25 as a mixed number and as an improper fraction.

The number 2.25 is read *two and twenty-five hundredths* and is written $2\frac{25}{100}$. You can simplify:

$$2\frac{25}{100} = 2\frac{\overset{1}{\cancel{25}}}{\underset{4}{\cancel{100}}} = 2\frac{1}{4}$$

$$= \frac{2 \times 4 + 1}{4} = \frac{9}{4}$$

So, 2.25 can be written as the mixed number $2\frac{1}{4}$ or as the improper fraction $\frac{9}{4}$.

$$\frac{25 \div 25}{100 \div 25} = \frac{1}{4}$$

In Example 1.5, $\frac{25}{100}$ was simplified by dividing both numerator and denominator by 25. This process is called **cancelling**.

Changing fractions to decimal numbers

To change a fraction to a decimal, as you would do in e.g. converting $^1/_2$ a litre of water to 0.5 L, think of the fraction as a division problem. For example:

$$\frac{2}{5} \quad \text{means} \quad 2 \div 5 \quad \text{or} \quad 5\overline{)2}$$

Here are the steps of the division.

Step 1   Replace 2 with 2.0 and then place a decimal point directly above the decimal point in 2.0:

$$5\overline{)2.0}^{\,\cdot}$$

Step 2   Perform the division:

$$\begin{array}{r} 0.4 \\ 5\overline{)2.0} \\ \underline{2\,0} \\ 0 \end{array}$$

So, $\frac{2}{5} = \underline{0.4}$.

Example 1.6

Write $\frac{193}{10}$ as a decimal number.

$$\frac{193}{10} \quad \text{means} \quad 193 \div 10 \quad \text{or} \quad 10\overline{)193}$$

Step 1 $\qquad\qquad 10\overline{)193.0}^{\,\cdot}$

Step 2
$$\begin{array}{r} 19.3 \\ 10\overline{)193.0} \\ \underline{10} \\ 93 \\ \underline{90} \\ 30 \\ \underline{30} \\ 0 \end{array}$$

So, $\frac{193}{10} = \underline{19.3}$.

There is a quicker way to do this problem. To divide a decimal number by 10, you move the decimal point in the number *one place to the left*. Notice that there is one zero in the 10:

$$\frac{193}{10} = \frac{193.}{10} = 19\,3. = 19.3$$

To divide a number by 100, move the decimal point in the number *two places to the left* because there are two zeros in 100. So, the quick way to divide by 10, 100, 1000, and so on is to count the zeros and then move the decimal point to the left the same number of places. The answer should always be a smaller number than the original number. Check your answer to be sure.

Stop and think

Fractions are written with one number over another – these are the numerator (top number) and denominator (bottom number). A patient requests some information from you – they have been told to decrease their salt intake by a quarter (1/4) to fit in with UK daily nutritional intake. They generally consume 2400 mg sodium (salt). You calculate this to be a reduction of 600 mg (2400 divided by 4 multiplied by 1) making an intake of 2400 minus 600 = 1800 mg. The challenge then is to work out what food they eat which will add up to the 600 mg they must reduce by.

Rounding decimal numbers

Sometimes it is convenient to round an answer – that is, to use an approximate answer rather than an exact one. This can be a process of 'rounding up' or 'rounding down' – the generally accepted convention is that numbers are rounded up or down to one or two decimal places.

Rounding numbers (up or down)

To round 1.267 *to the nearest tenth* – that is, to round off the number to one decimal place – do the following:

+ Look at the digit after the tenths place (the hundredths place digit).
+ Because this digit (6) is 5 or more, round up 1.267 by adding 1 to the tenths place digit.
+ Finally drop all the digits after the tenths place. So, 1.267 is approximated by 1.3 when rounded up to the nearest tenth.

To round off 0.8345 *to the nearest hundredth* – that is, to round off the number to two decimal places – do the following:

+ Look at the digit after the hundredths place (the thousandths place digit).
+ Because this digit (4) is less than 5, round down 0.8345 by leaving the hundredths digit alone.
+ Finally drop all the digits after the hundredths place. So, 0.8345 is approximated by 0.83 when rounded to the nearest hundredth.

Example 1.7

Round off 4.8075 to the nearest hundredth, tenth and whole number.

4.8075 rounded off to the nearest: hundredth = <u>4.81</u>

                                          tenth = <u>4.8</u>

                 whole number = <u>5</u>

To round *down* a number to a particular place, merely *drop all the digits after that place*. In particular, to round down to the tenths place, merely drop all the digits after the tenths place.

Example 1.8

Round down 4.8075 to the nearest hundredth, tenth and whole number.

4.8075 rounded *down* to the nearest: hundredth = <u>4.80</u>

                                        tenth = <u>4.8</u>

                 whole number = <u>4</u>

Practice point

The danger of an overdose must always be guarded against. Therefore, the amount of medication to be administered must not be rounded off or rounded down, most particularly in paediatrics or elderly care.

Multiplying and dividing decimal numbers

To multiply two decimal numbers, first multiply, ignoring the decimal points. Then count the total number of decimal places in the original two numbers. That sum equals the number of decimal places in the answer. Unless otherwise specified, quantities less than 1 will generally be rounded to the nearest hundredth, whereas quantities greater than 1 will generally be rounded to the nearest tenth.

Example 1.9

$$304.2 \times 0.16 = ?$$

304.2 ← 1 decimal place } Total of 3
× 0.16 ← 2 decimal places } decimal places

18252

3042
48.672

There are 3 decimal places in the answer.
Place the decimal point here.

So, $304.2 \times 0.16 = \underline{48.672}$.

11

Example 1.10

$$304.25 \times 10 = ?$$

$$
\begin{array}{r}
304.2\underline{5} \quad \leftarrow 2 \text{ decimal places} \\
\times\ 10 \quad \leftarrow 0 \text{ decimal places} \\
\hline
3042.\underline{50}
\end{array}
\left.\begin{array}{l} \\ \\ \end{array}\right\} \begin{array}{l} \text{Total of 2} \\ \text{decimal places} \end{array}
$$

There are 2 decimal places in the answer.
Place the decimal point here.

So, $304.25 \times 10 = \underline{3042.50}$ or $\underline{3042.5}$.

In Example 1.10 you can also use the rule of moving the decimal point (multiplying by 10). To multiply any decimal number by 10, move the decimal point in the number being multiplied *one place to the right*. Notice that there is one zero in 10:

$$304.25 \times 10 = 304.25 \quad \text{or} \quad 3042.5$$

To multiply a number by 100, move the decimal point in the number *two places to the right* because there are two zeros in 100. So, the quick way to multiply by 10, 100, 1000, and so on is to count the zeros and then move the decimal point to the right the same number of places. The answer should always be a larger number than the original. Check your answer to be sure.

Multiplying and dividing fractions

To multiply fractions, multiply the *numerators* to get the new numerator and multiply the *denominators* to get the new denominator.

Multiplication

Example 1.11

$$\frac{3}{5} \times 6 \times \frac{1}{5} = ?$$

A whole number can be written as a fraction with 1 in the denominator. So, in this example, write 6 as $\frac{6}{1}$ to make all the numbers fractions:

$$\frac{3}{5} \times \frac{6}{1} \times \frac{1}{5} = \frac{3 \times 6 \times 1}{5 \times 1 \times 5}$$

$$= \frac{18}{25}$$

Division

Example 1.12

$$1\frac{2}{5} \div \frac{7}{9} = ?$$

Write $1\frac{2}{5}$ as the improper fraction $\frac{7}{5}$. The *division* problem

$$\frac{7}{5} \div \frac{7}{9}$$

becomes the *multiplication* problem by inverting (turning around) the second fraction:

$$\frac{7}{5} \times \frac{9}{7}$$

$$\frac{\overset{1}{\cancel{7}}}{5} \times \frac{9}{\underset{1}{\cancel{7}}} = \frac{9}{5} = 1\frac{4}{5}$$

Sometimes you must deal with whole numbers, fractions, and decimal numbers in the same multiplication and division problems. *Avoid cancelling decimal numbers. It is a possible source of error.*

Example 1.13

Give the answer to the following problem in simplified fractional form:

$$\frac{1}{300} \times 60 \times \frac{1}{0.4} = ?$$

Write 60 as a fraction and cancel:

$$\frac{1}{\underset{5}{\cancel{300}}} \times \frac{\overset{1}{\cancel{60}}}{1} \times \frac{1}{0.4} = \frac{1}{5 \times 0.4} = \frac{1}{2}$$

Sometimes you will need to simplify *fractions that contain decimal numbers.*

Example 1.14

Give the answer to the following problem in simplified fractional form:

$$0.35 \times \frac{1}{60} = ?$$

Write 0.35 as the fraction $\frac{0.35}{1}$:

$$\frac{0.35}{1} \times \frac{1}{60} = \frac{0.35}{60}$$

The numerator of this fraction is 0.35, a decimal number. You can write an equivalent form of the fraction by multiplying the numerator and denominator by 100:

$$\frac{0.35}{60} \times \frac{100}{100} = \frac{35}{6000} = \frac{7}{1200}$$

Note

A useful rule of thumb – simplify the calculation before attempting it, this will avoid confusion. Always check your answers.

Complex fractions

Fractions that have numerators or denominators that are themselves fractions are called **complex fractions**.

The longest line in the complex fraction separates the numerator (top) from the denominator (bottom) of the complex fraction. As with any fraction, you can write the complex fraction as a division problem [*top ÷ bottom*].

In the complex fraction $\frac{1}{\frac{2}{5}}$, the numerator is 1 and the denominator is $\frac{2}{5}$. You can simplify this complex fraction as follows:

$$\frac{1}{\frac{2}{5}} \quad \text{means} \quad 1 \div \frac{2}{5} \quad \text{or} \quad 1 \times \frac{5}{2}, \quad \text{which is} \quad \frac{5}{2}$$

In the complex fraction $\frac{\frac{1}{2}}{5}$, the numerator is $\frac{1}{2}$ and the denominator is 5. You can simplify this complex fraction as follows:

$$\frac{\frac{1}{2}}{5} \quad \text{means} \quad \frac{1}{2} \div 5 \quad \text{or} \quad \frac{1}{2} \times \frac{1}{5}, \quad \text{which is} \quad \frac{1}{10}$$

In the complex fraction $\frac{\frac{3}{5}}{\frac{2}{5}}$, the numerator is $\frac{3}{5}$ and the denominator is $\frac{2}{5}$. You can simplify this complex fraction as follows:

$$\frac{\frac{3}{5}}{\frac{2}{5}} \quad \text{means} \quad \frac{3}{5} \div \frac{2}{5} \quad \text{or} \quad \frac{3}{\overset{}{5}} \times \frac{\overset{1}{5}}{2}, \quad \text{which is} \quad \frac{3}{2}$$

Example 1.15

$$\frac{\dfrac{1}{25} \times 500}{\dfrac{1}{4}} = ?$$

In this complex fraction, the numerator is $(\frac{1}{25} \times 500)$ and the denominator is $\frac{1}{4}$. So, you can write the following:

$$\left(\frac{1}{25} \times \frac{500}{1}\right) \div \frac{1}{4} = ?$$

Do the multiplication inside the brackets:

$$\left(\frac{1}{\cancel{25}} \times \frac{\cancel{500}^{20}}{1}\right) \div \frac{1}{4} =$$

$$\frac{20}{1} \div \frac{1}{4} =$$

$$\frac{20}{1} \times \frac{4}{1} = \underline{80}$$

Example 1.16

$$\frac{\dfrac{2}{3} \times \dfrac{1}{3}}{\dfrac{4}{}} = ?$$

You can multiply the numerators to get the new numerator and multiply the denominators to get the new denominator, as follows:

$$\frac{\dfrac{2}{3} \times \dfrac{1}{3}}{\dfrac{4}{}} = \frac{2 \times 1}{3 \times \dfrac{3}{4}} = \frac{2}{\dfrac{9}{4}}$$

Now, the numerator is 2 and the denominator is $\frac{9}{4}$, so you get

$$\frac{2}{1} \div \frac{9}{4}$$

which becomes

$$\frac{2}{1} \times \frac{4}{9} = \frac{8}{9}$$

This problem could have been done another way by simplifying $\dfrac{\dfrac{1}{3}}{\dfrac{3}{4}}$ first.

You can write $\dfrac{1}{\frac{3}{4}}$ as $1 \div \dfrac{3}{4}$. Then:

$$\dfrac{2}{3} \times \dfrac{1}{\frac{3}{4}} = \dfrac{2}{3} \times \left(1 \div \dfrac{3}{4}\right)$$

$$\dfrac{2}{3} \times \left(1 \times \dfrac{4}{3}\right)$$

$$\dfrac{2}{3} \times \left(\dfrac{4}{3}\right) = \underline{\dfrac{8}{9}}$$

Stop and think

Calculating with numbers in percent form can be difficult, so percentages should be converted to either fractional or decimal form before performing any calculations.

Percentages

Percent (%) means *parts per 100* or *divided by 100*. Thus 50% means 50 *divided by 100*, which can also be written as the fraction $\frac{50}{100}$. The fraction $\frac{50}{100}$ can be changed to the decimal numbers 0.50 and 0.5 or reduced to the fraction $\frac{1}{2}$.

13%   means $\dfrac{13}{100}$ or   0.13

100%   means $\dfrac{100}{100}$ or   1

12.3% means $\dfrac{12.3}{100}$ or   0.123

$6\dfrac{1}{2}\%$ means   6.5%   or $\dfrac{6.5}{100}$ or   0.065

Example 1.17

Write 0.5% as a fraction in lowest terms:

$$0.5\% = \dfrac{0.5}{100} = \dfrac{5}{1000} = \underline{\dfrac{1}{200}}$$

There is another way to get the answer. Because you understand that $0.5 = \frac{1}{2}$, then:

$$0.5\% = \dfrac{1}{2}\% = \dfrac{1}{2} \div 100 = \dfrac{1}{2} \div \dfrac{100}{1} = \dfrac{1}{2} \times \dfrac{1}{100} = \dfrac{1}{200}$$

Summary

In this chapter, all the essential mathematical skills that are used in this textbook were reviewed.

+ Addition, subtraction, division, etc. are known as mathematical operators.
+ The order of mathematical operators and functions can be remembered with the acronym: BODMAS (Brackets, Other, Division, Multiplication, Addition and Subtraction).
+ Three basic rules when attempting calculations: use common sense and estimation first, work out answers mentally, use appropriate formulas, and then lastly, check with a calculator.

When working with fractions

+ Any number can be changed into a fraction by writing the number over 1.
+ Proper fractions have smaller numbers in the numerator than in the denominator.
+ Improper fractions have numerators that are larger than or equal to their denominators.
+ Improper fractions can be changed to mixed numbers, and vice versa.
+ Cancel first when you multiply fractions.
+ Change a fraction to a decimal number by dividing the numerator by the denominator.
+ Simplify complex fractions by dividing the numerator by the denominator.

When working with decimals

+ Move the decimal point 3 places to the right when multiplying a decimal number by 1000.
+ Move the decimal point 3 places to the left when dividing a decimal number by 1000.
+ Count the total number of places in the numbers you are multiplying to determine the number of decimal places in the answer.
+ Avoid cancelling with decimal numbers.

When working with percentages

Change to fractions or decimal numbers before doing any calculations.

References

Hutton M (2005) Paediatric nursing calculation skills. *Paediatric Nursing* **17**(2): 1–17.

Kendrick A H and Smith E C (1992) Respiratory measurements. 2: Interpreting simple measurements of lung function. *Professional Nurse* **7**(11): 748, 750–2, 754.

Nursing and Midwifery Council (NMC) (2007) *Standards for Medicines Management*. London: Nursing and Midwifery Council.

Pierce R, Steinle V, Stacey K and Widjaja W (2008) Understanding decimal numbers: a foundation for correct calculations. *International Journal of Nursing Education Scholarship*: **5**(1). Available at: http://www.bepress.com/ijnes/vol5/iss1/art7 (accessed march 2009).

Case study 1.1

Calculation errors are a common occurrence in practice but particularly in paediatrics as the doses used vary according to the child's body weight. This quotation was taken from the Department of Health report 'Building a safer NHS for patients: Improving Medication Safety' – A report by the Chief Pharmaceutical Officer in 2003.

Death of a premature baby as a result of a morphine overdose
A junior doctor miscalculated a dose of intravenous morphine resulting in the administration of a 100 times overdose. The dose was calculated as 0.15 milligrams, but the decimal point was inserted in the wrong place and a dose of 15 milligrams was prescribed. The dose was administered to a premature baby who tragically died despite treatment with the antidote, naloxone.

The moral here is: **if in doubt ASK for help and ALWAYS double check calculations.**

Source: from *Building a Safer NHS for Patients: Improving Medication Safety – A Report by the Chief Pharmaceutical Officer*, Crown (2003), Crown copyright. Crown copyright material is reproduced with the permission of the Controller of HMSO and the Queen's Printer for Scotland.

Reflection

What can go wrong? In many areas of your life you frequently use calculations such as those outlined in this chapter and yet do not panic about them. Take time out to think about the following tasks – what would you do?

Task: You are cooking a celebratory meal for 6 people yet the recipe you have is for 24 people. What volume of ingredients will you require? What are the consequences if you do not alter the recipe? What type of numbers are involved?

Answer: This is an example of FRACTIONS. Since the numerator is 24 and the denominator is 6, thus $\frac{24}{6} = 4$. You require one part of that so the fraction is: 1/4 of the ingredients for your desired meal. The major consequences are that you cook too much food wasting money and time cooking (or have the same packed lunch for several days!!).

Task: There is a sale in your favourite shop – it is rather an expensive shop, but a sale is irresistible. You want some items, but there are two offers: today only it is *Buy TWO Get ONE Free*; or tomorrow it will be: *40% OFF*. You think about this – they seem so good! What types of numbers are these and which is the best deal? What is the worst that can happen?

Answer: The numbers can be FRACTIONS or DECIMALS – convert them to the same type of number to see which is the best deal. Thus: Buy two get one free means: you get 3 so one is free and you pay for 2 only or 1/3rd is free (which can also be written as 1 ÷ 3 which is 0.33 or to make it a percentage multiply by 100 so you get 33% off!). The 40% off deal is the better one! The worst that can happen is you buy too many items and waste money.

Task: A patient is prescribed 3.5 mg of a drug for pain relief. If the decimal point is missed then the patient could receive 35 mg of the drug. How much of an overdose would this be? What would the consequences be? What type of numbers are involved?

Answer: This is an example of DECIMALS. The patient would receive 10 times the prescribed drug. The patient has received an overdose, which is a drug error with potentially fatal consequences.

1. How did you feel about the non-clinical examples?

_____

2. How did you feel about the clinical example?

_____

List your concerns and identify how you can prepare to address these concerns and so gain confidence and competence:

1. _____
2. _____
3. _____
4. _____
5. _____

How will you know when you have improved? Make it measurable and specific!

Practice sets

The answers to *Try these for practice* and *Exercises* appear in Appendix A at the back of the book.

Try these for practice

Test your comprehension after reading the chapter.

1. Write $\frac{5}{16}$ as a decimal number. _____

2. Write $\frac{6.47 \times 2.3}{0.2}$ as a decimal number rounded off to the nearest tenth. _____

3. Write 40% as a decimal number and as a fraction in lowest terms. _____

4. $\frac{3}{7} \times \frac{14}{15} \times \frac{5}{6} =$ _____

5. Simplify: $\dfrac{\frac{5}{6}}{\frac{5}{12}}$ _____

Exercises

Reinforce your understanding in class or at home.

Convert to proper fractions or mixed numbers.

1. $0.85 =$ _____

2. $2.7 =$ _____

3. $40 \times \frac{1}{2} \times \frac{9}{16} =$ _____

4. $2\frac{3}{5} \div 2 =$ _____

5. $15 \div 3\frac{2}{3} =$ _____

6. $9.6 \div \frac{3}{7} =$ _____

7. $42 \times \frac{1}{9450} \times \frac{3}{0.02} =$ _____

Convert to decimal numbers.

8. $\frac{1}{8} =$ _____
(round down to the nearest hundredth)

9. $\frac{14}{25} =$ _____

10. $5\frac{3}{10} =$ _____

11. $\frac{1}{200} =$ _____

12. $\frac{1}{75} =$ _____
(round off to the nearest hundredth)

13. $\frac{870}{1000} =$ _____

14. $\dfrac{2.73}{100} =$ _____

15. $\dfrac{14.36}{7} =$ _____
(round down to the nearest tenth)

16. $\dfrac{0.63}{0.9} =$ _____

17. $\dfrac{0.063}{0.09} =$ _____

18. $5\dfrac{1}{2}\% =$ _____

19. $55\% =$ _____

Simplify and write the answer in decimal form.

20. $4.63 \times 6.21 =$ _____
(round off to the nearest hundredth)

21. $0.004 \times 100 =$ _____

22. $2.3456 \times 1000 =$ _____
(round off to the nearest tenth)

23. $850 \div 0.03 =$ _____

24. $8.5 \div 0.12 =$ _____
(round down to the nearest hundredth)

Simplify and write the answer in fractional form and in decimal form rounded off to the nearest tenth.

25. $0.72 \times \dfrac{1}{0.7} =$ _____

26. $\dfrac{\frac{2}{3}}{8} =$ _____

27. $\dfrac{\frac{2}{5}}{100} \times \dfrac{500}{6} =$ _____

28. $\dfrac{26 \times \frac{5}{13}}{\frac{9}{100}} =$ _____

29. $10.3\% =$ _____

30. $99.5\% =$ _____

Chapter 2

Safe and accurate drug administration

Learning outcomes

After completing this chapter, you will be able to

1. Describe the six rights of safe medication administration.
2. Explain the legal implications of medication administration.
3. Describe the routes of medication administration.
4. Identify common abbreviations used in medication administration.
5. Compare the proprietary (trade) names and non-proprietary (generic) name of drugs.
6. Describe the forms in which medications are supplied.
7. Identify and interpret the components of a drug prescription.
8. Interpret the information found on drug labels and drug package inserts.

This chapter introduces the process of safe and accurate medication administration. The rights of the patients and the responsibilities of the people involved in the administration of medication are described.

As patients may receive medications in a variety of forms, these various forms and routes of drugs are presented as well as abbreviations used in prescribing and documenting the administration of medications. You will learn how to interpret drug prescriptions, drug labels, medication administration records and package inserts. You may wish to refer to a good-quality pharmacology book on seeing some of the drug examples that will be used in this chapter and subsequent chapters, as pharmacological explanations are not provided (no space or scope in this text). The examples are used to illustrate the main points (names, labels, forms).

Diagnostic questions

Before commencing this chapter try to answer the following questions. Compare your answers with those in Appendix A in order to identify your strengths and areas to focus on.

1. What is a drug prescription?

_____

2. Who are the main people involved in the prescription process?

_____

3. How many RIGHTS of drug administration are there?

_____

4. What is the role of a drug package insert?

_____

5. What does the GENERIC name of a drug mean?

_____

The drug administration process

Drug administration is a process involving a chain of healthcare professionals. The **prescriber writes** the drug prescription, the **pharmacist dispenses** the prescription and the **nurse or other healthcare professional administers** the drug to the patient; each is responsible for the accuracy of the prescription. The legal responsibility for the pre-scription lies with the person who signs the prescription (DoH 2008). Furthermore, there are a range of professional and non-healthcare individuals (e.g. in residential institutions, etc., including patients themselves) who may administer drugs.

To ensure patient safety, knowledge of how drugs act and interact in patients is import-ant either for one's own practice or for education, support and guidance of patients and colleagues. Drugs can be life-saving or life-threatening. Every year, thousands of deaths occur because of medication errors. Errors can occur at any point in the medication process from prescribing to dispensing or administration (Smith 2004).

Who administers drugs?

There are a range of healthcare professionals who can prescribe drugs from general practitioners, hospital doctors, pharmacist independent prescribers, optometrist inde-pendent prescribers, dentists and other independent prescribers (DoH 1999, 2008). Some nurse practitioners can also prescribe following qualification as independent prescribers. There are two groups of independent nurse prescribers: Community Practitioner Nurse Prescribers, who qualified under the original arrangements for nurse prescribing, and Nurse Independent Prescribers (PPD 2008). In 2005 the Department of Health announced a wider range of health professionals who could prescribe under a category called: _Supplementary prescribers_, doing so in association with a doctor (DoH 2008).

Although prescribers may administer drugs to patients, other professionals, namely **registered nurses, midwives** and **specialist community nurses,** are usually responsible for administering drugs. In some situations, designated non-professional personnel administer drugs or medications to clients (residential homes), and this is generally following training and preparation for competence whilst also following local policies and maintaining strict records of administration (RPSGB 2003).

Healthcare professionals who administer drugs or medications must be familiar with their professional body guidance. For nurses this is: the Nursing and Midwifery Council (NMC) Standards for Medicines Management (2007). Furthermore, healthcare professionals do need to be aware of specific local policies and procedures relative to the administration of medications, and that they have a legal and ethical responsibility to report medication errors. There are many organisations and groups that are striving to reduce medication errors, such as the Medicines and Healthcare products Regulatory Agency (MHRA), National Patient Safety Agency (NPSA), the Department of Health (DoH), National Institute for Health and Clinical Excellence (NICE), the Royal College of Nursing (RCN) and the NMC mentioned above. Professionals have a responsibility to be aware of their limitations and work towards addressing these with colleagues, workplace, professional bodies, education institutions and also resources such as this book.

Note

A generic drug may be manufactured by different companies under different trade names. For example, the generic drug ibuprofen is manufactured by Abbott McNeil PPC under the trade name Brufen, and by Reckitt Benckiser plc Wyeth pharmaceuticals under the trade name Nurofen. The active ingredients in Brufen and Nurofen are the same, but the size, shape, colour or fillers may be different. Be aware that patients may become confused and worried about receiving a medication that has a different name or appears to be dissimilar from their usual medication.

Practice point

The person who administers the drug has the last opportunity to identify an error before a patient might be injured or harmed. Rigorous checking should not be ignored even if it has already been done!

Six rights of medication administration

In order to prepare and administer drugs, it is imperative that you understand and follow professional guidance (NMC 2007) and focus on the *six rights of medication administration* (Figure 2.1):

+ right drug
+ right dose
+ right route
+ right time
+ right patient
+ right documentation

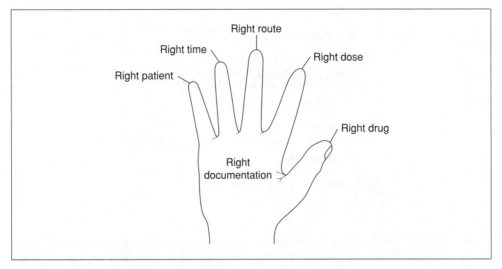

Figure 2.1 Six rights of drug administration

These six 'rights' should be checked before administering any medications. Failure to achieve any of these rights constitutes a medication error.

Some institutions or clinical areas recognise additional rights, such as the **right to know**, the **right to refuse** and the **right attitude**. Patients need to be informed and educated about their medications as they are a partner in their care and treatment. If a patient refuses a medication, the reason must be documented and reported immediately.

The right drug

A drug is a chemical substance that acts on the physiological processes in the human body. For example, the drug insulin is given to patients whose pancreas cannot produce insulin. Some drugs have more than one action. Aspirin, for example, is an antipyretic (fever-reducing), analgesic (pain-relieving) and anti-inflammatory drug that also has anti-coagulant properties (keeps the blood from clotting). A drug may be taken for one, some or all its therapeutic properties.

The **generic** or **non-proprietary** name is the official accepted name of a drug, as listed in the British National Formulary (BNF). A drug has only one non-proprietary name, but can have many proprietary or trade names. By law, the European Union (EU) directive on labelling of medicines 92/27/EEC *requires the use of recommended international non-proprietary names (rINN) for drugs.*

In many instances the British Approved Name (BAN) and the rINN were identical; where they were not, the BAN was modified to comply for consistency and safety (BNF 2008). Many companies may manufacture the same drug using different proprietary (**trade**, **patented** or **brand**) names. The drug's proprietary name is followed by the **trademark** symbol ™ or the **registration** symbol ®. For example, **Avodart**® is the proprietary name and **dutasteride** is the non-proprietary name for the drug shown in Figure 2.2. **Dosage strength** indicates the amount of drug in a specific unit of measurement. The dosage strength of Avodart is 0.5 mg per capsule.

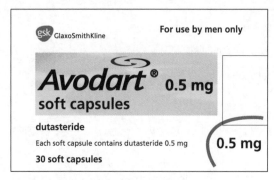

Figure 2.2 Drug label for Avodart

(Reproduced with the permission of GlaxoSmithKline)

To help avoid errors, drugs should be prescribed using only the non-proprietary name. There are also economic implications. Proprietary brands and sophisticated or colourful packaging may cost more than simpler plain non-proprietary brands of drugs. This may require extra vigilance by the nurse or whoever is administering the drug or even the patient who may be self administering. Do note that *some drugs have names that sound alike, or have names or packaging that look similar, thus a working knowledge of the names is essential. If in doubt always consult a pharmacological text such as the BNF or the Electronic Medicines Compendium (EMC) or ask the local pharmacist.* Table 2.1 includes a sample list of drugs whose names may be confused.

Practice point

Patients may become confused with drug packaging changes, so it is important that the nurse understands the concepts of proprietary and non-proprietary forms of drugs and can advise, explain and support patients self-administering drugs to minimise anxiety and potential errors. There is a move to make the design of drug packaging and labels clearer, but patients still require support (NPSA 2007).

Table 2.1 Look-alike/sound-alike drugs

Drug name	Look-alike/sound-alike drug name
ceftazidime	cefotaxime
dactinomycin	daptomycin
ephedrine	epinephrine
fluconazole	fluorouracil
folic acid	folinic acid
Humalog	Humulin
hydralazine	hydroxyzine
nizatidine	nifedipine
Retrovir	ritonavir
vinblastine	vincristine

Stop and think

Giving the wrong drug is a common medication error. In order to avoid errors, carefully read drug labels at the following times, even if the dose is pre-packaged, labelled and ready to be administered:

+ when reaching for the container;
+ immediately before preparing the dose;
+ when replacing or discarding the container.

These are referred to as the *three checks*.

Always question the patient concerning any allergies to medications! Make sure the drug is not expired, and never give a drug from a container that is unlabelled or has an unreadable label.

Practice point

The calibrated dropper *supplied with a medication* should be used ONLY for that medication. For example, the dropper that is supplied with digoxin (Lanoxin) cannot be used to measure furosemide (Lasix).

The right dose

A person prescribing or administering medications has the **legal responsibility** of knowing the correct dose. Since no two people are exactly alike, and no drug affects every human body in exactly the same way, drug doses must be individualised. Responses to drug actions differ according to the gender, race, genetics, nutritional and health status, age, and weight of the patient (especially children and the elderly), as well as the route and time of administration.

Body surface area (BSA) is an estimate of the total skin area of a person measured in metres squared (m^2). Body surface area is determined by formulas based on height and weight or by the use of a BSA nomogram (see Chapter 5). Many drug doses administered to children or used for cancer therapy are calculated based on BSA.

Before administering drugs to patients there are some essential steps to take:

+ Carefully read the drug label to determine the **dosage strength**.
+ Perform and *check calculations* and pay special attention to decimal points.
+ When giving an IV drug to a paediatric patient or giving a high-alert drug (one that has a high risk of causing injury), always *double check the dosage and if using a pump, the pump settings*, and confirm these with a colleague according to your local policy. Be aware that many institutions or clinical areas may operate a single checking policy.
+ Be sure to check for the recommended *safe dosage range* based on the patient's age, BSA or weight.
+ After you have calculated the dose, be certain to administer using standard measuring devices such as calibrated medicine droppers, syringes or cups.

The right route

Medications must be *in the form* and *via the route specified by the prescriber*. Medications are manufactured in a variety of forms: tablets, capsules, liquids, suppositories, creams, patches or injectable medications (which are supplied in solution or in a powdered form to be reconstituted). The route indicates the site of entry into the body and method of drug delivery.

Oral medications

Oral medications are administered **by mouth** (PO). Oral drugs are supplied in both solid and liquid form.

+ The most common solid forms are *tablets* (tab), *capsules* (cap) and *caplets* (Figure 2.3).

+ **Scored** tablets have a groove down the centre so that the tablet can be easily broken in half. To avoid an incorrect dose, unscored tablets should never be broken for administration (Lister 2008).

+ **Enteric-coated** tablets are meant to dissolve in the intestine rather than in the stomach. Therefore, they should be neither chewed nor crushed.

+ A **capsule** contains a powder, liquid or granules in a gelatin case. *Sustained-release* (SR) or *extended-release* (XR) tablets or capsules slowly release a controlled amount of medication into the body over a period of time. Therefore, these drugs should not be opened, chewed or crushed.

+ Tablets for *buccal* administration (absorbed by the mucosa of the mouth) and tablets for *sublingual* (SL) administration (absorbed under the tongue) should never be swallowed.

+ Oral drugs also come in liquid forms: *elixir*, *syrup* and *suspension*. An **elixir** is an alcohol solution, a **syrup** is a medication dissolved in a sugar and water solution and a **suspension** consists of an insoluble drug in a liquid base.

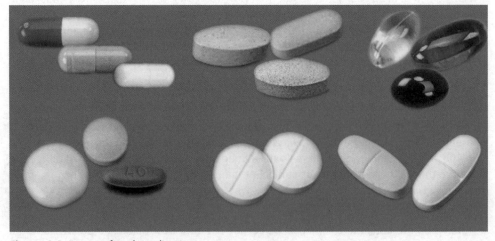

Figure 2.3 Forms of oral medications

Practice point

> *DO NOT* substitute a different route for the prescribed route because a serious over-dose or underdose may occur. Drug forms are made specifically for particular routes so tablets or capsules cannot be used for parenteral or injectable routes.

Parenteral medications

Parenteral medications are those that are injected (via needle) into the body by various routes. Drug forms for parenteral use are sterile and must be administered using aseptic (sterile) technique. The most common parenteral sites are the following:

+ **intramuscular (IM):** into the muscle;
+ **subcutaneous (subcut):** into the subcutaneous tissue;
+ **intravenous (IV):** into the vein;
+ **intradermal (ID):** beneath the skin.

Cutaneous medications

Cutaneous medications are those that are administered through the skin or mucous membrane. Cutaneous routes include the following:

+ **topical:** administered on the skin surface;
+ **transdermal:** contained in a patch or disk and applied to the skin;
+ **inhalation:** breathed into the respiratory tract through the nose or mouth;
+ **solutions and ointments:** applied to the mucosa of the eyes (optic), nose (nasal), ears (otic) and mouth;
+ **suppositories:** shaped for insertion into a body cavity (vagina or rectum) and dissolve at body temperature.

Some drugs are supplied in multiple forms and therefore can be administered by a variety of routes. For example, Voltarol (Novartis) (diclofenac sodium) is supplied as a tablet, dispersible tablet, suppository, topical gel or solution for injection.

The right time

The prescriber will indicate when and how often a medication should be administered. Oral medications can be given either before or after meals, depending on the action of the drug. Medications can be prescribed *once a day* (daily/od), *twice a day* (b.i.d./bd), *three times a day* (t.i.d./tds) and *four times a day* (q.i.d./qds). Most health or clinical institutions indicate specific times for these administrations. To maintain a more stable level of the drug in the patient, the administration of the drug should be prescribed for regular intervals, such as every 4 hours, 6 hourly or 12 hourly.

It should be noted that the term b.i.d. (twice daily) is not necessarily the same as 12 hourly. B.i.d. may mean administer at 10 A.M. and 6 P.M., whereas 12 hourly may mean *administer at 10 A.M. and 10 P.M.* (depending on the particular local institutional policy). Drugs can also be prescribed to be administered as needed (*pro re nata* or prn).

29

Stop and think

Timing of medication administration can be critical for maintaining a stable concentration of the drug in the blood and avoiding interactions with other drugs. Usually a dose should be given within 30 minutes of the time specified by the prescriber – up to 30 minutes before or 30 minutes after. For some medications this could be disastrous; for example, giving insulin too early with a time delay until a meal may result in a patient having a low blood sugar episode (hypoglycaemia) which could be dangerous. In addition, be aware of professional responsibilities: it is imperative that the patient is observed taking the drug; if it is left to take 'later' this constitutes negligence – once the administration process is commenced the steps should be followed *all* the way through.

Know the local policy and always administer the dose directly after it is prepared.

The right patient

Before administering any medication, it is essential to determine the identity of the recipient. The NMC clearly states in standard 8 of the Standards for Medicines Management (2007) that 'you must be *certain* of the identity of the patient to whom the medication is to be administered.' To be certain you must check:

+ **Verbally**: ask the patient their name, date of birth, if an in-patient also the hospital number, if known.
+ **Visually**: check the patient name band (if in-patient) against the name on the prescription chart.
+ *Never use the patient's bed number or room number*. After identifying the patient, match the prescription chart, patient's name, age and hospital number or address.

The right documentation

Always check the prescription form for the correct legible name and dosage of the drug, as well as the route and time of administration. If one is being used also ensure the Medication Administration Record (MAR) is clearly completed and signed. Sign your initials *immediately after, but never before*, the dose is given. It is important to document any relevant information in the patient's care plan. For example, document patient allergies to medications, specific measurement, e.g. heart rate (when giving digoxin) or blood pressure (when giving antihypertensive drugs). All documentation must be legible. Remember the old saying, 'If it's not documented, it's not done.'

Anticipate side effects! A side effect is an undesired physiological response to a drug. For example, codeine relieves pain, but its side effects include constipation, nausea, drowsiness and itching. A nurse or whoever is administering the drug must be sure to record any observed side effects and discuss them with the prescriber.

Safe drug administration requires a knowledge of common abbreviations. For instance, when the prescriber writes *'Pethidine 75 mg IM 4 hourly prn pain'*, the person administering the drug reads this as *'Pethidine, 75 milligrams, intramuscularly, every four hours, as needed for pain'*. Only approved abbreviations should be used (Table 2.2).

Table 2.2 Common abbreviations used for medication administration

Abbreviation	Meaning	Abbreviation	Meaning
Route:		qqh	quarta quaque hora (every four hours)
ID	intradermal	om or mane	omni mane (every morning)
IM	intramuscular		
IV	intravenous	on or nocte	omni nocte (every night)
IV bolus	intravenous bolus	prn	pro re nata (when required)
NG	nasogastric tube		
PEG	percutaneous endoscopic gastrostomy	Stat	immediately
PO	by mouth	**General:**	
PR	by rectum	cap	capsule
SL	sublingual	ER	extended release
Supp	suppository	g	gram
		h, hr	hour
Frequency:		kg	kilogram
ac	ante cibum (before food)	L	litre
pc	post cibum (after food)		
od	omni die (every day)	mg	milligram
bd	bis die (twice daily)	mL	millilitre
tds	ter die sumendum (to be taken three times daily)	NBM	nil by mouth
		NKA	no known allergies
tid	ter in die (three times daily)	SR	sustained release
qds	quater die sumendum (to be taken four times daily)	Susp	suspension
		tab	tablet

Drug prescriptions

Before anyone can administer any medication, there must be a legal prescription for the medication.

A **drug prescription** is a directive for a drug to be given to a patient and is based on patient consent to the treatment, recently more commonly known as a **patient specific directive**. In order for a patient to receive a drug which is paid for by the NHS a particular prescription must be completed (FP10). Some medicines are normally only available on prescription and not surprisingly these are referred to as prescription only medicines (or POMs). In addition, patients receive products on prescription that are not licensed medicinal products, for example appliances or dressings. Other medicines can be bought in pharmacies or from general retail outlets, and this is a consideration for nurses when administering medications to patients to avoid situations of administering medications and patients self-administering their own purchased medication at the same time.

Patients who are an in-patient in a hospital will have medications prescribed on hospital prescription charts for use during the in-patient period only. These charts will be devised by and be specific for the local hospital to fulfil its requirements and possibly any specific speciality. As nurses move from hospital to hospital or between differing clinical areas they may become confused with the differing drug prescription charts and need to be familiar with the key aspects of them and their own specific responsibilities. Hospital in-patient prescription charts differ from the legal standard NHS FP10 prescription forms (FP10s). The hospital doctor may prescribe some medication to take away on discharge home (TTAs) on these, generally for a short period, but these are not routinely used in hospital situations.

The standard NHS FP10 prescription forms are available in a variety of formats so different types of prescribers use their own specific versions of this form. Each version is a different colour, which helps the dispenser and the Prescription Pricing Division to identify the prescriber's profession. The different versions of the FP10 also have different codes to indicate the type of prescriber authorised to prescribe, e.g. Nurses – FP10P, FP10SS, FP10 MDA-SS.

Information necessary for inclusion is listed below.

+ Further information.
+ Date the prescription is written.
+ For in-patient prescriptions include: the patient's full name, date of birth and hospital number.
+ Drug name (generic name should be used preferably), dosage, route, frequency and amount to be dispensed (i.e. duration of therapy – 5 days or 1 month, etc.).
+ Allergies or previous drug sensitivities (adverse drug reactions).
+ Number of refills permitted.

When writing and checking prescriptions one should also adhere to the following as advised by the BNF (2008) and Smith (2004):

+ Unnecessary use of decimal points should be avoided, e.g. 5 mg, not 5.0 mg.
+ Quantities less than 1 gram should be written in milligrams, e.g. 500 mg, not 0.5 g.
+ Quantities less than 1 mg should be written in micrograms, e.g. 100 micrograms, not 0.1 mg.
+ When decimals are unavoidable a zero should be written in front of the decimal point where there is no other figure, e.g. 0.5 mL, not .5 mL.
+ Micrograms and nanograms should **not** be abbreviated. Similarly units should **not** be abbreviated.

If the prescriber has an objection to a generic drug substitute, the prescriber will write 'do not substitute,' 'dispense as written,' 'no generic substitution,' or 'medically necessary.' (Figure 2.4).

PHARMACY STAMP:	AGE: *17*	NAME (INCLUDING FORENAME) AND ADDRESS: *Peter Patient* *Flat 1, 50 Stanhope Street* *Newtown TE22 1ST*			
	D.O.B *02/04/1992*	NHS NUMBER: *QT 123*			
DISPENSER'S ENDORSEMENT	NUMBER OF DAYS TREATMENT. N.B ENSURE DOSE IS STATED		NP		PRICING OFFICE
PACK & QUANTITY	*Amoxycillin 125 mg (syrup)* *PO 3 times a day for 7 days* *Complete the course of medication*				
SIGNATURE OF DOCTORS *Dr. D.O. Good*				DATE: *02/07/2009*	
FOR DISPENSER NO. OF ITEMS ON FORM	DOCTOR ADDRESS AND TELEPHONE NUMBER: *7 High Street* *Any Town KB1 CD2* *0111 222 333*				
PLEASE READ NOTES OVERLEAF					

Figure 2.4 Drug prescription for Amoxycillin

Directions to the patient for use maybe included, but this will be clearly identified by the pharmacist dispensing the drug or medication following NPSA guidance. This prescription is interpreted as follows:

Prescriber:	*Dr D O Good*
Prescriber address:	*7 High Street, Anytown, KB1 CD2*
Prescriber phone number:	*0111 222 333*
Date prescription written:	*02/07/2009*
Patient full name:	*Mr Peter Patient*
Patient address:	*Flat 1, 50 Stanhope Street, Newtown, TE22 1ST*
Patient date of birth:	*02/04/1992*
Drug name:	*Amoxycillin*
Dosage:	*125 mg*
Route:	*PO*
Frequency:	*Three times a day*
Amount to be dispensed:	*7 days worth*
Directions to the patient:	*Take 125 mg three times a day for 7 days. Ensure the course is completed.*
Refill instructions:	*No more refills on this prescription.*

Example 2.1

Read the prescription in Figure 2.5 and complete the following information.

PHARMACY STAMP:	AGE: 46	NAME (INCLUDING FORENAME) AND ADDRESS: *Maria Silvestri* *124 Windy Lane* *Old Town* *WD4 6 BT*			
	D.O.B *11/07/63*	NHS NUMBER: *KT1111*			
DISPENSER'S ENDORSEMENT	NUMBER OF DAYS TREATMENT. N.B ENSURE DOSE IS STATED		NP		PRICING OFFICE
PACK & QUANTITY	*Doxcycline 100 mg* *PO B.D. for 7 days*				
SIGNATURE OF DOCTORS *A.J. Smith*				DATE: *10/01/09*	
FOR DISPENSER NO. OF ITEMS ON FORM	DOCTOR ADDRESS AND TELEPHONE NUMBER: *A.J. Smith* *1234 Spring Street* *Old Town WD9 7GB*				
PLEASE READ NOTES OVERLEAF					

Figure 2.5 Drug prescription for doxycycline

Date prescription written: _____

Patient full name: _____

Patient address: _____

Patient date of birth: _____

Generic drug name: _____

Dosage: _____

Route: _____

Frequency: _____

Amount to be dispensed: _____

Directions to the patient: _____

Refill instructions: _____

This is what you should have found:

Date prescription written:	10/01/09
Patient full name:	Maria Silvestri
Patient address:	124 Windy Lane, Old Town, WD4 6 BT
Patient date of birth:	11/07/63
Generic drug name:	Doxcycline
Dosage:	100 mg
Route:	PO (orally)
Frequency:	B.D. (twice daily)
Amount to be dispensed:	7 days worth
Directions to the patient:	Take 100 mg orally twice a day for 7 days.
Refill instructions:	None indicated.

Prescriptions and medication administration records

Prescription forms

Prescription forms are directives to the pharmacist for the drugs used in a hospital or other health institution. No medication should be given without a valid legible prescription form (FP10) or hospital-specific in-patient prescription chart. According to the standards set out by the NMC (2007) a verbal order on its own is not sufficient (Lister 2008). In exceptional circumstances medication – not including controlled drugs – which have been prescribed previously can be re-prescribed using information technology such as fax, text message or email. However, the changes must be followed up with a written prescription normally within 24 hours (72 hours maximum at weekends and bank holidays).

Stop and think

If persons administering drugs or medications have difficulty understanding, reading or interpreting the orders, they must clarify the orders with the prescriber. Consider the effect of administering Daonil (hypoglycaemic drug) instead of Amoxil (antibiotic) because the prescriber's handwriting was illegible.

A *verbal* order must contain the same components as a written order or else it is invalid. In order to provide for the safety of the patient, generally verbal orders may be taken only in an emergency. Each medication order should follow a specific sequence:

35

drug name, dose, route and frequency. The verbal order must be written and signed by the physician within 24 hours.

Prescription variations

The most common type of prescription is the *routine FP10 prescription* as mentioned before, which indicates the drug to be administered until discontinued, terminated (signed and dated) or until a specified date is reached. If an in-patient, the patient will have their medication prescribed on a specific hospital prescription developed and adapted for use in that particular area. Recording of administration of medications may also be on the same form; this will, however, vary in residential, community and out-patient areas and the nurse is advised to check on the documents in use.

A **prn** prescription is written by the prescriber for a drug to be given when a patient needs it; for example, '*Codeine 30 mg PO 4 hourly prn for mild to moderate pain.*'

A **stat** prescription is an order that is to be administered immediately. Stat orders are usually written for emergencies or when a patient's condition suddenly changes; for example, '*Lasix 80 mg IV stat*' for heart failure: Lasix to be given once immediately.

Other variations on a prescription chart may include specific sections for specific treatments and regimes, e.g. there may be a prophylaxis section – products or medications to prevent a problem occurring such as heparin medication or anti-embolic stockings. Regimes which need to be evaluated and assessed frequently may have particular sections on in-patient prescription charts, e.g. insulin administration, anticoagulation, oxygen therapy or intravenous infusions. The nurse should be familiar with all aspects and specifics of medication prescription and associated administration demands.

Following recent changes and developments, prescriptions can take the form of conventional prescription sheets completed by a doctor or other trained and prepared prescriber (also called non-medical independent prescribing and supplementary prescribing) on forms discussed above. Another variation is a Patient Group Direction (PGD) or a Clinical Management Plan (CMP). Patient Group Directions are documents which make it legal for medicines to be given to groups of patients – for example in a clinic (family planning, etc.) situation – without individual prescriptions having to be written for each patient. They are not prescriptions but locally agreed written instructions signed by a doctor and a pharmacist and approved by the healthcare body (NMC 2007). They allow some qualified nurses to administer named medications to specific groups of patients with particular clincial conditions (Lister 2008). They can also be used to empower staff other than doctors (for example paramedics and nurses) to legally give the medicine in question (DoH 2008; NPC 2004).

Components of a prescription

The essential components of a prescription are the following (Figure 2.6):

+ **Patient's full name and date of birth:** This information can be printed on a label attached to the prescription form. Additional information may include the patient's admission number, religion and consultant or general practitioner (family doctor) name.

+ **Date and time the prescription was written:** This includes the month, day, year and time of day. Many institutions use the '24 hour clock' for precision, that does not use

✚ GENERAL HOSPITAL ✚

PRESS HARD WITH BALLPOINT PEN. WRITE DATE &TIME AND SIGN EACH ITEM

DATE	TIME	A.M.
20/11/2009	*0800h*	P.M.

IMPRINT
602412   20/11/09
John Camden   11/2/55
23 Jones Avenue   RC
Anytown BT 45 9AB

Dr I. Patel

Captopril 25 mg PO t.i.d. for 7 days

PRESCRIPTION NOTED

DATE *20/11/09* TIME *0830*   A.M.
                                P.M.

NURSE'S SIG. *Mary Jones RN*

FILLED BY   DATE

SIGNATURE

Dr I. Patel

IN-PATIENT PRESCRIPTION

Figure 2.6 Drug prescription for captopril

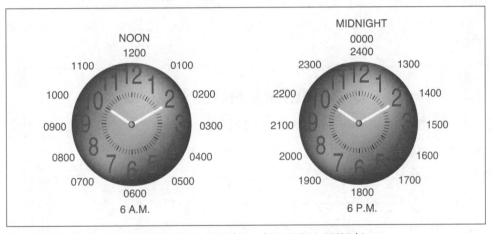

Figure 2.7 Clocks showing 10:10 A.M. (1010 h) and 10:10 P.M. (2210 h)

A.M. or P.M. (Figure 2.7). The 24 hour clock times are written as four-digit numbers. Thus, 2:00 A.M. is 0200 h, 12 noon is 1200 h, 2:00 P.M. is 1400 h and midnight is 2400 h, also written as 0000 h.

+ **Name of the medication:** The generic name is recommended. If a prescriber wants to prescribe a trade name drug, 'no generic substitution' should be specified.

+ **Dosage of the medication:** The amount of the drug.

+ **Route of administration.**

+ **Time and frequency of administration.**

+ **Signature of the prescriber:** The prescription is not legal without the signature of the prescriber.
+ **Signature of the person administering the prescription:** This may be the responsibility of a nurse or others identified by local policy.

The in-patient prescription in Figure 2.6 can be interpreted as follows:

Name of patient:	*John Camden*
Birth date:	*11/02/1955*
Date of admission:	*20/11/2009*
Hospital Number:	*602412*
Religion:	*Roman Catholic (RC)*
Date and time the prescription was written:	*20/11/2009 at 0800 h or 8:00 A.M.*
Name of the medication:	*captopril*
Dosage:	*25 mg*
Route of administration:	*PO (by mouth)*
Frequency of administration:	*t.i.d., three times a day for 7 days*
Signature of person writing the prescription:	*Dr I Patel*
Person who administered the medication:	*Mary Jones, RN*

Example 2.2

Interpret the following prescription chart shown in Figure 2.8 and record the following information:

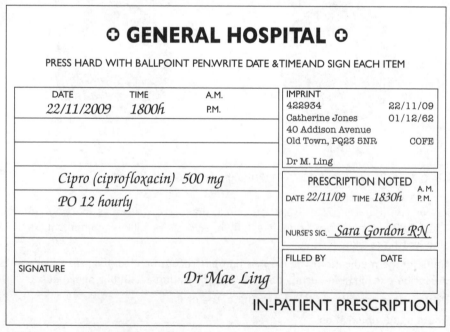

Figure 2.8 Drug prescription for Cipro

Date prescription written: _____

Time prescription written: _____

Name of drug: _____

Dosage: _____

Route of administration: _____

Frequency of administration: _____

Name of prescriber: _____

Name of patient: _____

Birth date: _____

Religion: _____

Person who administered the medication: _____

This is what you should have found:

Date prescription written:	*22/11/2009*
Time prescription written:	*1800 h or 6:00 P.M.*
Name of drug:	*ciprofloxacin*
Dosage:	*500 mg*
Route of administration:	*by mouth*
Frequency of administration:	*every 12 hours*
Name of prescriber:	*Dr Mae Ling*
Name of patient:	*Catherine Jones*
Birth date:	*01/12/1962*
Religion:	*Protestant*
Person who administered the medication:	*Sara Gordon, RN*

The **Clinical Management Plan (CMP)** is the foundation stone of supplementary prescribing by a non-medical practitioner. Before supplementary prescribing can take place, it is obligatory for an agreed CMP to be in place (written or electronic) relating to a named patient and to that patient's specific condition(s) to be managed by the supplementary prescriber. This should be included in the patient record.

It is essential that prescriptions should contain the following necessary elements (following the guidance from the British National Formulary):

+ Should be written legibly in ink or otherwise so as to be indelible.
+ Should be dated, should state the full name and address of the patient and should be signed in ink by the prescriber.

The age and the date of birth of the patient should preferably be stated, and it is a legal requirement in the case of prescription-only medicines to state the age for children under 12 years.

Medication administration records

Medication administration records are often used in homes and residential care institutions, which should also be referred to in association with the patient's prescription and care plan. A **Medication Administration Record (MAR)** is a form that some healthcare institutions and other areas such as care homes and residential institutions increasingly use to document all the drugs administered to a patient. It is important to note that nurses or anyone else routinely administering medication should be prepared and informed of the responsibilities of drug and medicine administration. Invariably, non-professional colleagues will administer oral or topical medications, as injectable or other routes require specific training.

The national minimum standard for all care homes is set by the Care Home Regulations (2001, cited in CSCI 2008) is that the records detail for each person:

+ what is received;
+ what is currently prescribed (including those self-administering medicines);
+ what is given by care workers;
+ what is disposed of.

Routine, **PRN** and **STAT medications** all may be written in separate locations on the MAR. If a medication is to be given regularly, a complete schedule is written for all administration times. Each time a dose is administered, the person administering the medication initials the time of administration. The initials of the person who gave the medication must be recorded on the MAR. However, a record of the full name, title and initials of all persons administering medication should be maintained in the patient's care plan, especially in a long-term care institution where only designated persons can administer the medications.

This should not be confused with prescription sheets but recognised as a record of medication administration. After the prescription has been verified, a nurse or other healthcare worker administers the medication. The MAR may be used to check the prescription, prepare the correct medication dose and record the date, time and route of administration.

The essential components of the MAR include the following:

+ **Patient information:** a printed label with patient identification (name, date of birth, hospital number). If a printed label is not available this may be hand-written in block capitals.
+ **Dates:** when the prescription was written, when to start the medication and when to discontinue it.
+ **Medication information:** full name of the drug, dose, route and frequency of administration.

+ **Time of administration:** frequency as stated in the prescriber's prescription; for example, t.i.d. Times for prn and *one-time doses* are recorded *precisely* at the time they are administered.

+ **Initials:** the initials and the signature of the person who administered the medication are recorded.

+ **Special instructions:** instructions relating to the medication; for example, 'Omit if systolic BP is less than 100.'

Example 2.3

Study the MAR in Figure 2.9 then complete the following chart and answer the questions.

Name of drug	Dose	Route of administration	Time of administration

1. Identify the drugs and their doses administered at 9:00 A.M.

2. Identify the drugs and their doses administered at 9:00 P.M.

3. What is the route of administration for famotidine?

4. What is the time of administration for famitodine?

UNIVERSITY HOSPITAL	789652 Wendy Kim 44 Chester Avenue London N23 6BB	09/12/09 20/12/60 RC
DAILY MEDICATION ADMINISTRATION RECORD	Dr John Rodriguez	

PATIENT NAME ___*Wendy Kim*___

ROOM ___*422*___   IF ANOTHER RECORD IS IN USE ☐

ALLERGIC TO (RECORD IN RED): ___*tomato, codeine*___

				TIME:	DATE:		
DRUG: *Famotidine*					*09/12/09*	*10/12/09*	*11/12/09*
ROUTE: *Po*	DOSE: *20 mg*	START DATE: *09/12/2009*	STOP DATE: *18/12/2009*	*06.00*	*X*	*JY*	
SIGNATURE:		ADDITIONAL INSTRUCTIONS:		*18.00*	*JY*	*JY*	
PHARMACY/STOCK							

DRUG: *Digoxin*					*09/12/09*	*10/12/09*	*11/12/09*
ROUTE: *PO*	DOSE: *0.125 mg*	START DATE: *09/12/2009*	STOP DATE: *18/12/2009*	*09.00*	*JY*		
SIGNATURE:		ADDITIONAL INSTRUCTIONS:					
PHARMACY/STOCK		*Once daily at same time*					

DRUG: *Captopril*					*09/12/09*	*10/12/09*	*11/12/09*
ROUTE: *PO*	DOSE: *25 mg*	START DATE: *09/12/2009*	STOP DATE: *18/12/2009*	*09.00*	*JY*	*JY*	
SIGNATURE:		ADDITIONAL INSTRUCTIONS:		*21.00*	*JY*	*JY*	
PHARMACY/STOCK							

DRUG: *Alprazolam*					*09/12/09*	*10/12/09*	*11/12/09*
ROUTE: *PO*	DOSE: *0.5 mg*	START DATE: *09/12/2009*	STOP DATE: *18/12/2009*				
SIGNATURE:		ADDITIONAL INSTRUCTIONS:					
PHARMACY/STOCK				*21.00*	*JY*	*JY*	

Figure 2.9 MAR for Wendy Kim

This is what you should have found:

Name of drug	Dose	Route of administration	Time of administration
famotidine	20 mg	PO	0600 h (6 A.M.) and 1800 h (6 P.M.)
digoxin	0.125 mg	PO	0900 h (9 A.M.)
captopril	25 mg	PO	0900 h (9 A.M.) and 2100 h (9 P.M.)
alprazolam	0.5 mg	PO	2100 h (9 P.M.)

1. Digoxin 0.125 mg; captopril 25 mg.

2. Captopril 25 mg; alprazolam 0.5 mg.

3. PO.

4. 0600 h (6 A.M.) and 1800 h (6 P.M.).

Computerised recordkeeping

In the future many health institutions or areas may computerise the medication process; at present this is sometimes seen at family doctors or general practitioner practices. Those who prescribe or administer medications must use security codes and passwords to access the computer system. Prescribers input information regarding prescriptions and all other essential patient information directly into a computer terminal. The prescription is received in the pharmacy, where a patient's drug profile (list of drugs) is maintained. A computer printout replaces the handwritten prescription.

One advantage of a computerised system is that handwritten orders do not need to be deciphered or transcribed. The computer program can also identify possible interactions among the patient's medications and automatically alert the pharmacist and persons administering the drugs. However, until this is widespread, human error may occur and attention to detail with the drug or medication administration process is crucial.

Drug labels

You will need to read, interpret and understand the information found on drug labels in order to calculate drug dosages. There are several important features of a drug label, and the Medicines and Healthcare Products Regulatory Agency (MHRA 2003) published best practice guidance for drug labels and drug package inserts or patient information leaflets (PiLs) in response to the concerns by the Department of Health and Chief Medical Officers for patient safety.

As part of a wider initiative to reduce medication errors, the Committee on Safety of Medicines (CoSM) reviewed the factors that are involved in labelling and packaging and, as a result of their work, agreed the principles that should be used when labelling medicines. The main objective was to make improvements to medicines labelling within the current regulatory framework, to assist healthcare professionals and patients/carers to select the correct drug or medicine and use it safely, thereby helping to minimise medication errors.

Labelling must contain *all* elements required by article 54 of Council Directive 2001/83/EEC (MHRA 2003: 5). Nevertheless, certain items of information are deemed critical for the safe use of the medicine. These items are:

+ **name of the medicine**
+ **strength of the medicine/drug** (where relevant)
+ **route of administration**
+ **posology** (pharmacological information about appropriate doses of drugs)
+ **specific warnings** (not for IV use or dilute with water).

There is also guidance on font type and size so that critical information should be in as large a font as possible to maximise legibility. For further information refer to MHRA guidance.

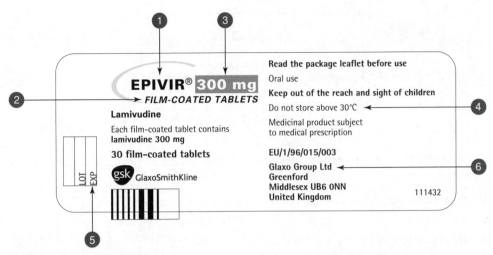

Figure 2.10 Drug label for Epivir

(Reproduced with the permission of GlaxoSmithKline)

The label for Epivir in Figure 2.10 indicates the following:

1. **Name of drug:** Epivir is the trade name. In this case, the name is in large type and is boldly visible on the label. The generic name is Lamivudine (rINN name).

2. **Form of drug:** The drug is in the form of a tablet.

3. **Dosage strength:** 300 mg of the drug are contained in one tablet.

4. **Storage directions:** Some drugs have to be stored under controlled conditions if they are to retain their effectiveness. This drug should be stored below 30°C.

5. **Expiration date:** The expiration date specifies when the drug should be discarded. For the sake of simplicity, not every drug label in this textbook will have an expiration date.

6. **Manufacturer:** Glaxo Group.

Practice point

Always read the expiration date! This is important because, after the expiration date, the drug may lose its potency or act differently in a patient's body. Expired drugs should be discarded either in the clinical area or given to the pharmacy for disposal. Never give expired drugs to patients and patients should be advised not to keep drugs for a long time 'just in case' as they will not be as effective.

> Metoprolol tartrate
> 50 mg tablets
> Expiry December 2010
> Protect from moisture
> Dispense in tight, light-resistant
> container

Figure 2.11 Drug label for metoprolol tartrate

The label for the antihypertensive drug metoprolol tartrate in Figure 2.11 indicates the following:

1. **Generic name:** *metoprolol tartrate*
2. **Form:** *tablets*
3. **Dosage strength:** *50 mg per tablet*
4. **Expiration:** *discard after 31/12/10*
5. **Instructions for dispensing:** *protect from moisture and dispense in tight, light-resistant container.*

Example 2.4

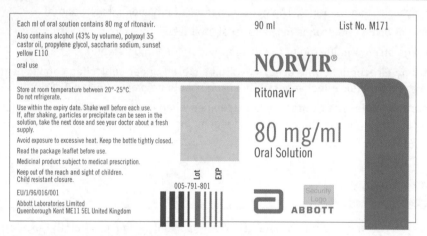

Figure 2.12 Drug label for Norvir

(Reproduced with permission of Abbott Laboratories)

Examine the label shown in Figure 2.12 and record the following information:

1. Trade name: _____

2. Generic name: _____

3. Form: _____

4. Dosage strength: _____

5. Amount of drug in container: _____

6. Storage temperature: _____

7. Special instructions: _____

This is what you should have found:

1. **Trade name:** *Norvir*
2. **Generic name:** *ritonavir*
3. **Form:** *oral solution*
4. **Dosage strength:** *80 mg per mL*
5. **Amount of drug in container:** *90 mL*
6. **Storage temperature:** *at room temperature, between 20°C – 25°C*
7. **Special instructions:** *shake well before use. Keep out of reach of children.*

Drug package inserts

Sometimes information needed to safely prepare, administer and store medications is not located on the drug label. In such cases, you may need to read the **summary of product characteristics (SPC)** or the **Patient Information Leaflet (PiL)**. SPCs are used by health-care professionals and explain how to use and prescribe a medicine. SPCs are written and updated by pharmaceutical companies, based on their research and product knowledge. The PiL is also written by the pharmaceutical company and is a patient-friendly version of the SPC. SPCs and PiLs are checked and approved by the UK or European medicines licensing agency. Figure 2.13 shows an excerpt from the PiL for Avodart.

Avodart® 0.5 mg soft capsules dutasteride

WHAT AVODART IS AND WHAT IT'S USED FOR

Avodart is used to treat men with an enlarged prostate *(benign prostatic hyperplasia)* – a non-cancerous growth of the prostate gland, caused by producing too much of a hormone called dihydrotestosterone. The active ingredient is dutasteride. It belongs to a group of medicines called 5-alpha reductase inhibitors. As the prostate grows, it can lead to urinary problems, such as difficulty in passing urine and a need to go to the toilet frequently. It can also cause the flow of the urine to be slower and less forceful. If left untreated, there is a risk that your urine flow will be completely blocked *(acute urinary retention)*. This requires immediate medical treatment. In some situations surgery is necessary to remove or reduce the size of the prostate gland. Avodart lowers the production of dihydrotestosterone, which helps to shrink the prostate and relieve the symptoms. This will reduce the risk of acute urinary retention and the need for surgery.

Avodart may also be used with another medicine called tamsulosin (used to treat the symptoms of an enlarged prostate).

HOW TO TAKE AVODART

Always take Avodart exactly as your doctor has told you to. Check with your doctor or pharmacist if you are not sure.

How much to take
- **The usual dose is one capsule (0.5 mg) taken once a day.**
  Swallow the capsules whole with water. Do not chew or break open the capsule. Contact with the contents of the capsules may make your mouth or throat sore.
- Avodart is a long term treatment. Some men notice an early improvement in their symptoms. However, others may need to take Avodart for 6 months or more before it begins to have an effect. Keep taking Avodart for as long as your doctor tells you.

Figure 2.13 Excerpts from Avodart package insert

(Reproduced with the permission of SmithGlaxoKline. See http://emc.medicines.org.uk for full text)

Figure 2.13 (*continued*)

If you take too much Avodart

Contact your doctor or pharmacist for advice if you take too many Avodart capsules.

If you forget to take Avodart

Don't take extra capsules to make up for a missed dose. Just take your next dose at the usual time.

Don't stop Avodart without advice

Don't stop taking Avodart without talking to your doctor first. It may take up to 6 months or more for you to notice an effect.

If you have any further questions on the use of this product, ask your doctor or pharmacist.

POSSIBLE SIDE EFFECTS

Like all medicines, Avodart can cause side effects, although not everybody gets them.

Very rare allergic reaction

The signs of allergic reactions can include:

- **skin rash** (which can be itchy)
- **hives** (like a nettle rash)
- **swelling of the eyelids, face, lips, arms or legs.**

→ **Contact you doctor immediately** if you get any of these symptoms, and **stop using Avodart**.

Common side effects

These may affect up to 1 in 10 men taking Avodart:

- impotence *(not able to achieve or maintain an erection)*
- decreased sex drive *(libido)*
- difficulty with ejaculation
- breast enlargement or tenderness *(gynecomastia)*
- dizziness when taken with tamsulosin.

→ If any of the side effects gets serious, or if you notice any side effects not listed in this leaflet, please tell your doctor or pharmacist.

HOW TO STORE AVODART

Keep out of the reach and sight of children.

Don't store Avodart above 30°C.

Don't use Avodart after the expiry date which is stated on the carton or the foil blister strip. The expiry date refers to the last day of that month.

If you have any unwanted Avodart capsules, don't dispose of them in waste water or household rubbish. Take them back to your pharmacist, who will dispose of them in a way that won't harm the environment.

FURTHER INFORMATION

What Avodart contains

The active substance is dutasteride. Each soft capsule contains 0.5 mg dutasteride.

The other ingredients are:

- inside the capsule: mono and diglycerides of caprylic/capric acid and butylated hydroxytoluene (E321).
- capsule shell: gelatin, glycerol, titanium dioxide (E171), iron oxide yellow (E172), triglycerides (medium chain), lecithin
- printed ink: iron oxide red (E172) as the colourant, polyvinyl acetate phthalate, propylene glycol and macrogol.

What Avodart looks like and contents of the pack

Avodart soft capsules are oblong opaque, yellow, soft gelatin capsules printed with GX CE2 on one side in red ink. They are available in packs of 30 capsules.

Marketing Authorisation Holder

GlaxoSmithKline UK
Stockley Park West
Uxbridge
Middlesex
UB11 1BT

Manufacturer:

Catalent France Beinheim SA
74 rue Principale
67930 Beinheim
France

Always consult the package information insert when you need information about:

+ mixing and storing a drug
+ preparing a drug dose
+ recommended safe dose and range
+ indications, contraindications, and warnings
+ side effects and adverse reactions

Example 2.5

Read the package insert for Avodart in Figure 2.13 and fill in the requested information:

1. What is the generic name of the drug?

_____

2. For what condition is Avodart (dutasteride) used?

_____

3. How long after Avodart (dutasteride) has been started might a patient wait for effects?

_____

4. What is the recommended dose of the drug?

_____

5. What is the drug form?

_____

This is what you should have found:

1. Dutasteride.
2. Benign prostatic hyperplasia (BPH).
3. Men being treated with dutasteride may not see results until 6 months have passed.
4. The recommended dose of Avodart (dustaseride) is 1 capsule (0.5 mg) orally once a day.
5. The drug is supplied in the form of soft gelatin capsules.

Summary

In this chapter, the Medication Administration Process was discussed, including those who may administer drugs; the 'six rights' and 'three checks' of medication administration; how to interpret prescriptions and medication administration records, drug labels and drug package inserts.

How to administer drugs

+ The six rights of medication administration serve as a guide for **safe** administration of medications to patients.

+ Failure to achieve any of the six rights constitutes a medication error.

+ A person administering medications has a legal, ethical and moral responsibility to report medication errors.

+ Medication errors can occur at any point in the medication process.

+ A drug should be prescribed using its generic name.

+ Understanding drug orders requires the interpretation of common abbreviations.

+ Read drug labels carefully; many drugs have look-alike/sound-alike names.

+ Carefully read the label to determine dosage strength and check calculations, paying special attention to decimal points.

+ Medications must be administered in the form and via the route specified by the prescriber.

+ Before administering any medication, it is essential to identify the patient.

+ Medications should be documented immediately after, but never before, they are administered.

+ No medication should be given without a prescription order.

+ If persons administering medications have difficulty understanding or interpreting the order, they must clarify the order with the prescriber.

+ Medication administration is rapidly becoming computerised.

+ Drug package inserts contain detailed information about the drug, including mixing, storing a drug, preparing a drug dose, indications, contraindications, warnings, side effects, adverse reactions and the recommended safe dose range.

+ If in doubt about any of the steps in the process do not administer the drug but seek expert help from the prescriber or pharmacist.

References

Commission for Social Care Inspection (CSCI) (2008) *Professional Advice: Medicine administration records (MAR) in care homes and domiciliary care*. QPM document 124/08. London: Commission for Social Care inspection.

Department of Health (DoH) (1998) *Review of Prescribing, supply and administration of medicines. A Report of the supply and administration Group Protocols*. London: HMSO.

Department of Health (DoH) (1999) *Review of Prescribing, supply and administration of medicines Final Report*. London: HMSO.

Department of Health (DoH) (2008) Supplementary Prescribing. Available from http://www.dh.gov.uk/en/Healthcare/Medicinespharmacyandindustry/Prescriptions/TheNon-MedicalPrescribingProgramme/Supplementaryprescribing/index.htm, accessed March 2009.

Joint Formulary Committee (BNF) (2008) *British National Formulary (55)*. London: British Medical Association and Royal Pharmaceutical Society of Great Britain.

Lister S (2008) *Drug Administration General Principles*. In Doughty L and Lister S (eds) *The Royal Marsden Hospital Manual of Clinical Nursing Procedures*, 7th edition. Oxford: Wiley-Blackwell Publishing.

Medicines and Healthcare Regulatory Agency (MHRA) (2003) *Best practice guidance on labelling and packaging of medicines. Guidance Note No. 25*. London: Medicines and Healthcare Products Regulatory Agency.

National Patient Safety Agency (NPSA) (2007) *Design for Patient Safety: a guide to the design of dispensed medicines*. London: National Patient Safety Agency/National Health Service.

National Prescribing Centre (NPC) (2004) *Patient Group Directions; A practical guide and framework of competencies for all professionals using patient group directions*. Liverpool: National Prescribing Centre. Available at: http://www.npc.co.uk/publications/pgd/pgd.pdf (accessed March 2009).

Nursing and Midwifery Council (NMC) (2007) *Standards for Medicines Management*. London: Nursing and Midwifery Council. Available at: http://www.nmc-uk.org/aDisplayDocument.aspx?DocumentID=3251 accessed March 2009.

Prescription Pricing Division (2008) *Prescribers and FP10 prescriptions*. Newcastle upon Tyne: NHS Business Services Authority. Available at: http://www.nhsbsa.nhs.uk/PrescriptionService/1865.aspx (accessed March 2009).

Royal Pharmaceutical Society of Great Britain (RPSGB) (2003) *The Administration and Control of Medicines in Care Homes and Children's Services*. London: Royal Pharmaceutical Society of Great Britain.

Smith J (2004) *Building a Safer NHS for Patients: Improving Medication Safety*. London: HMSO.

Practice sets

The answers to *Try these for practice* and *Exercises* appear in Appendix A at the end of the book.

Try these for practice

Test your comprehension after reading the chapter.

Study the drug labels in Figures 2.14 to 2.17 and answer the following four questions.

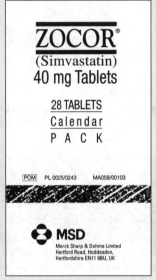

Figure 2.14 Drug label for Zocor
(From Merck Sharp & Dohme Ltd, reproduced with permission)

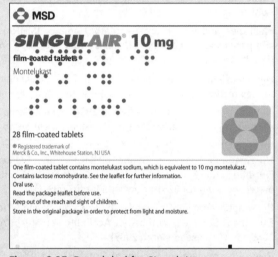

Figure 2.15 Drug label for Singulair
(Reproduced with permission, Merck Sharp & Dohme Ltd)

Imatinib mesilate
400 mg tablets

Figure 2.16 Drug label for imatinib mesilate

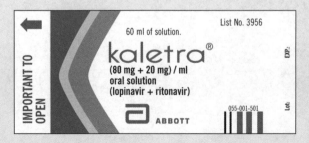

Figure 2.17 Drug label for Kaletra
(Reproduced with permission of Abbott Laboratories)

1. What is the route of administration for montelukast sodium?

   _____

2. How many tablets are contained in the container for Zocor?

   _____

3. What is the tablet dose of imatinib mesylate?

   _____

4. What is contained in 1 mL of the drug Kaletra?

   _____

Exercises

Reinforce your understanding in class or at home.

Use the information from drug labels in Figures 2.14 to 2.17 to complete the following two exercises.

1. Write the generic name for Kaletra.

   _____

2. What is the dosage strength of Zocor?

   _____

3. Study the Medicine Administration Record for Jane Ambery in Figure 2.18. Fill in the following chart and answer the questions.

   (a) Which drugs were administered at 10 P.M. on 10/12/09?

   _____

   (b) Designate the time of the day the patient received ibandronic acid.

   _____

   (c) How many doses of phenytoin were administered to the patient by nurse Young?

   _____

   (d) What drugs must be taken before breakfast?

   _____

   (e) What is the last date on which the patient will receive Trimethoprim?

   _____

324689
Jane Ambery
17 Magnolia Avenue
Brighton BT23

07/12/09
9/05/47
COFE

Dr Mae Ling

UNIVERSITY HOSPITAL

DAILY MEDICATION ADMNISTRATION RECORD

PATIENT NAME _Jane Ambery_

WARD _Rose_

ALLERGIC TO (RECORD IN RED): _fish_

IF ANOTHER RECORD IS IN USE ☐

DATES GIVEN ↓ MONTH/DAY   YEAR: _2009_

				TIME:	DATE:		
DRUG: *Phenytoin*					09/12/09	10/12/09	11/12/09
ROUTE: PO	DOSE: 100 mg	START DATE: 07/12/2009	STOP DATE:	10.00	MC	MC	MC
SIGNATURE: Dr Jones		ADDITIONAL INSTRUCTIONS:		14.00	MC	MC	MC
PHARMACY/STOCK				18.00	JY	JY	JY

					09/12/09	10/12/09	11/12/09
DRUG: *Trimethoprim*							
ROUTE: PO	DOSE: 100 mg	START DATE: 07/12/2009	STOP DATE: 18/12/2009	08.00	MC		
SIGNATURE: Dr Jones		ADDITIONAL INSTRUCTIONS: *For 10 days*		18.00	JY		
PHARMACY/STOCK							

					09/12/09	10/12/09	11/12/09
DRUG: *Ibandronic acid*							
ROUTE: PO	DOSE: 50 mg	START DATE: 07/12/2009	STOP DATE: 18/12/2009	06.00	JY	JY	
SIGNATURE: Dr Jones		ADDITIONAL INSTRUCTIONS: *Take 60 minutes before first food*					
PHARMACY/STOCK		*or drink in the morning*					

					09/12/09	10/12/09	11/12/09
DRUG: *Anusol*							
ROUTE: Rectal	DOSE: one	START DATE: 09/12/2009	STOP DATE:	22.00		JY	
SIGNATURE: Dr Jones		ADDITIONAL INSTRUCTIONS:					
PHARMACY/STOCK							

INT.	NURSES' FULL SIGNATURE AND TITLE	INT.	NURSES' FULL SIGNATURE AND TITLE
SG	Sara Gordon R.N.		
MC	Marie Colon R.N.		
JY	Jim Young R.N.		

Figure 2.18 MAR for Jane Ambery

4. Study the Prescription Chart for Jane Myers in Figure 2.19 and then answer the following questions.

PHARMACY STAMP:	AGE: 57	NAME (INCLUDING FORENAME) AND ADDRESS: *Jane Myers* *23 College Ave* *Anytown* *AT 555 9YY*			
	D.O.B *28/02/52*	NHS NUMBER: *BT 1234*			
DISPENSER'S ENDORSEMENT	NUMBER OF DAYS TREATMENT. N.B ENSURE DOSE IS STATED		NP		PRICING OFFICE
PACK & QUANTITY	*Cefalexin 500 mg PO 12 hourly for ten (10) days* *Digoxin 0.125 mg PO once daily* *Metformin 850 mg PO BD wtih breakfast and evening meal* *Metoclopramide 10 mg PO 30 minutes before meals and at bedtime* *Fentanyl transdermal patch 25 mg per hour. Remove afer 72 hours. one (1)* *Furosemide 40 mg PO once daily*				
SIGNATURE OF DOCTORS *A.J. Rodriguez*				DATE: *10/04/09*	
FOR DISPENSER NO. OF ITEMS ON FORM	DOCTOR ADDRESS AND TELEPHONE NUMBER: *A.J. Rodriguez* *1234 Hope Street* *Old Town WD9 7GB*				
PLEASE READ NOTES OVERLEAF					

Figure 2.19 Drug prescription for Jane Myers

(a) Which drugs are ordered to be given once daily?

_____

(b) Which drug should be given four times a day?

_____

(c) What is the dose and route of administration of metoclopramide?

_____

(d) What is the route of administration for fentanyl?

_____

(e) Which drug is given every 12 hours?

_____

5. Use the package insert shown for Diazepam in Figure 2.20 to answer the following questions.

(a) What is an appropriate dose for relief of children with muscle spasm?

_____

(b) Treatment should not usually exceed how long?

_____

(c) What is the dosage strength of the Diazepam Oral Solution?

_____

6. Fill in the following table with the equivalent times.

Standard time	24 hour clock
9 a.m.	_____
_____	1500 h
_____	1200 h
6 p.m.	_____
_____	2015 h
2:30 a.m.	_____
_____	1645 h
6 a.m.	_____
_____	0000 h

---

actavis

Diazepam Oral Solution 2mg/5ml

- Please read this leaflet carefully before you start to take your medicine.
- It gives you important information about your medicine.
- If you want to know more, or you are not sure about anything, ask your pharmacist or doctor.
- Keep the leaflet untit you have finished the medicine.

WHAT'S IN YOUR MEDICINE

Diazepam Oral Solution comes in one strength containing 2 mg of the active ingredient diazepam per 5 ml solution. It is a pink syrup with an odour of raspberries.

The solution also contains: docusate sodium, magnesium aluminium silicate, propylene glycol, raspberry flavour, saccharin sodium, erythrosine (E127), sorbic acid (E200), propyl hydroxybenzoate (E216), methyl hydroxybenzoate (E218), sorbitol (E420), glycerol (E422). Diazepam Oral Solution is available in a pack size of 100 ml.

Diazepam is one of a group of medicines called benzodiazepine tranquillisers. These medicines act on brain transmitters and help in the treatment of anxiety and muscle spasms.

MA holder: Actavis, Barnstaple, EX32 8NS, UK.
Manufacturer: Pinewood Laboratories Ltd,
Ballymacarbry, Clonmel, Ireland.

ABOUT YOUR MEDICINE

The name of your medicine is Diazepam Oral Solution which is the generic (common) name. Your doctor may have given you this medicine before from another company and it may have looked slightly different. Either brand will have the same effect.

Diazepam Oral Solution may be used:

- for the short term (2 weeks) relief of anxiety, which is severe, disabling, distressing and may be associated with sleeplessness or with other mental illnesses.
- to relieve muscle spasms in cerebral palsy, tetanus or other causes of muscular spasm.
- to relieve muscle weakness.
- to help in the treatment of certain forms of epilepsy (usually epilepsy associated with muscular spasms).
- to relieve the symptoms of acute alcohol withdrawal.
- as an oral pre-medication for nervous dental patients.
- in children with spasticity to control tension and irritability.
- as an oral pre-medication in children.

TAKING YOUR MEDICINE

Your doctor has decided the dose which is best for you. Always follow your doctor's instructions exactly, and those on the pharmacy label. If you do not understand anything ask your doctor or pharmacist.

The usual dosage(s) are described below.

Indication/Dosage

Anxiety, obsession & other mental illness:
2–30 mg (5–75 ml solution) daily in divided doses.

Anxiety associated with sleeplessness.
5–30 mg (12.5–75 ml solution) before going to bed.

Cerebral palsy:
2–60 mg (5–150 ml solution) daily in divided doses.

Other causes of muscle spasms:
2–60 mg (5–150 ml solution) daily in divided doses.

Epilepsy:
As a pre-medication 2–60 mg (5–150 ml solution) daily in divided doses.
In adults 5–20 mg (12.5–50 ml solution) daily.
In children 2–10 mg (5–25 ml solution) daily.

Alcohol withdrawal:
5–20 mg (12.5–50 ml solution), repeated if necessary in 2–4 hours.

Pre-medication in dental patients:
5 mg (12.5 ml solution) the night before treatment, 5 mg (12.5 ml solution) on waking and 5mg (12.5 ml solution) two hours before the appointment.

Elderly and debilitated patients:
Dose should be half the recommended doses.

Spastic children with a little amount of brain damage:
2–40 mg (5–100 ml solution) daily in divided doses.

Children with muscle spasms:
2–40mg (5–100 ml solution) daily in divided doses. If associated with tetanus the adult dose should be given.

If you are elderly, it is particularly important to take this medicine exactly as directed by the doctor.

This solution should be taken by mouth as instructed. Shake the bottle before use and make sure that the bottle is always kept tightly shut when not in use. Continue to take it for as long as your doctor tells you to, it may be dangerous to stop without their advice. Treatment should not usually exceed 2 weeks and should be gradually withdrawn as adverse effects, such as difficulty sleeping, irritability, nervousness, sweating, diarrhoea and depression, have been observed on abrupt withdrawal. If you forget to take a dose, take another as soon as you remember and then your next dose at the usual time. NEVER take two doses at the same time. If you accidentally take more than your prescribed dose, contact your nearest hospital casualty department, or tell your doctor, immediately. Take any remaining solution and the container with you.

STORING YOUR MEDICINE

Do not use the solution after the expiry date shown on the product packaging. Do not store above 25°C. Keep container in the outer carton and keep the container tightly closed. **KEEP IT IN A SECURE PLACE WHERE CHILDREN CANNOT GET AT OR SEE IT. REMEMBER**, this medicine is for **YOU** only. **NEVER** give it to anyone else. It may harm them, even if their symptoms are the same as yours. Unless your doctor tells you to, do not keep medicines that you no longer need – give them back to your pharmacist for safe disposal.

Date of last revision: January 2007

actavis
Actavis, Barnstaple, EX32 8NS, UK
3LF560

Figure 2.20 Excerpts from package insert for Diazepam

(Courtesy of Actavis. See http://emc.medicines.org.uk for full text)

Chapter 3

Changing units of measurements

Learning outcomes

After completing this chapter, you will be able to

1. Identify some common units of measurement and their abbreviations.

2. Construct fractions from decimals.

3. Convert a quantity expressed in one unit of measurement to an equivalent quantity with another unit of measurement.

4. Convert a quantity expressed as one rate to another different rate.

In this chapter you will learn how to convert measurements from one form to another. This will underpin all drug calculations and, whilst it may seem daunting, it can be mastered with a little practise. These skills are useful in all areas of life and work from catering for a party or function to converting a patient's daily drug dose to divided doses (three or four times) in a day.

Diagnostic questions

Before commencing this chapter try to answer these questions. Compare your answers with those in Appendix A in order to identify which aspects you need to focus on.

1. You are having a tea party with four of your colleagues at work. You have brought a small cake and cut it up equally between the four of you. What is another term for one portion of that cake?

2. One colleague is on a diet and so you eat two portions of the cake. What is another way of communicating this amount?

3. Mr Jones has a fluid restriction. One colleague tells you he has had $3/4$ of his allowance and another colleague tells you he has had 75%. Are these different amounts?

4. Which is the greater amount, 104 weeks or 2 years?

5. A patient must exercise 30 minutes twice a day. He tells you he prefers to exercise 10 minutes six times a day. Will he have enough exercise?

Introduction to units of measurement and conversions

In courses such as chemistry and physics, students learn to routinely change a quantity in one unit of measurement to an equivalent quantity in a different unit of measurement by cancelling matching units of measurement. Consider planning your annual leave; you may have 7 weeks holiday a year which works out as 35 days and you may be thinking about how you will use these days. Or you wish to work out which bank will give you the best interest rate – some advertise it monthly, others annually, and you need to convert them to the same so you can understand them and make a judgement. In clinical practice this will take on a different meaning but you will use similar skills, e.g. converting an intravenous fluid flow rate of a solution from litres per hour to millilitres per minute. To do this effectively it is necessary to practise using fundamental mathematical concepts, some of which build upon information in the previous chapters.

The mathematical foundation

This relies on two simple mathematical concepts.

Concept 1

When a nonzero quantity is divided by the same amount, the result is 1.

For example: $7 \div 7 = 1$

Because you can also write a division problem in fractional form, you get:

$$\frac{7}{7} = 1$$

Since $\frac{7}{7}$ is a fraction equal to 1, and the word 'unit' means one, the fraction $\frac{7}{7}$ is called a unit fraction.

In the preceding example, you may simplify or **cancel** the 7s on the top and bottom. That is, you can divide both numerator and denominator by 7:

$$\frac{\cancel{7}}{\cancel{7}} = \frac{1}{1} = 1$$

Units of measurement are the 'labels,' such as *centimetres, metres, kilograms, minutes* and *hours*, which are sometimes written after a number. They are also referred to as **dimensions**, or simply **units**. For example, in the quantity 7 *days, days* is the unit of measurement.

The equivalent quantities you divide may contain **units of measurement**.

For example: 7 days ÷ 7 days = 1

Or in fractional form

$$\frac{7 \text{ days}}{7 \text{ days}} = 1$$

In the preceding unit fraction, you may cancel the number 7 and the unit of measurement *days* on the top and bottom and obtain the following:

$$\frac{\cancel{7 \text{ days}}}{\cancel{7 \text{ days}}} = \frac{1}{1} = 1$$

Going one step further, now consider this **equivalence**: *7 days = 1 week*. Because *7 days* is the same quantity of time as 1 *week*, when you divide these quantities, you must get 1.

So, both 7 days ÷ 1 week = 1   *and*   1 week ÷ 7 days = 1

Or in unit fractional form

$$\frac{7 \text{ days}}{1 \text{ week}} = 1 \quad and \quad \frac{1 \text{ week}}{7 \text{ days}} = 1$$

Other unit fractions can be obtained from the equivalences found in Table 3.1.

Table 3.1 Equivalents for common units

1000 millilitres (mL) = 1 litre (L)	
60 seconds (sec)	= 1 minute (min)
60 minutes (min)	= 1 hour (h or hr)
24 hours (h or hr)	= 1 day (d)
12 months (mon)	= 1 year (yr)
16 ounces (oz)	= 1 pound (lb)

Concept 2

When a quantity (or number) is multiplied by 1, the quantity (or number) is unchanged.

In the following examples, the quantity *2 weeks* will be multiplied by the number 1 and also by the unit fractions $\frac{7}{7}$, $\frac{7 \text{ days}}{7 \text{ days}}$ and $\frac{7 \text{ days}}{1 \text{ week}}$.

2 weeks × 1 =   2 weeks

2 weeks × $\frac{7}{7}$ = 2 weeks × 1 = 2 weeks

2 weeks × $\frac{7 \text{ days}}{7 \text{ days}}$ = 2 weeks × 1 = 2 weeks

2 weeks × $\frac{7 \text{ days}}{1 \text{ week}}$ = 2 weeks × 1 = 2 weeks

Consider the previous line again. This time you cancel the *week(s)*, so all you end up with is the *unit of measurement you are interested in*:

$$2 \text{ weeks} \times \frac{7 \text{ days}}{1 \text{ week}} = 2 \text{ weeks} \times \frac{7 \text{ days}}{1 \text{ week}} = (2 \times 7) \text{ days} = 14 \text{ days}$$

So, 2 weeks = 14 days.

This shows how to convert a quantity measured in weeks (2 *weeks*) to an equivalent quantity measured in days (14 *days*). With this method, you will be multiplying quantities by unit fractions in order to convert the units of measure. Many of the problems in dosage calculation require changing a quantity with a *single unit of measurement* into an equivalent quantity with a different *single unit of measurement*; for example, changing 2 *weeks* to 14 *days* as was done above. Other problems may involve changing one type of *rates of flow (e.g. L/min)* to equivalent but different *rates of flow e.g. (mL/sec)*. Both of these types of problems will be addressed in this chapter.

Changing a single unit of measurement to another single unit of measurement

Simple problems with single units of measurement

Imagine you want to express 18 *months* in *years*. That is, you want to convert 18 *months* to an equivalent amount of time in *years*. This is a **simple** problem. Simple problems have only three elements. The elements in this problem are:

The given quantity:	18 months
The quantity you want to find:	? years
An equivalence between them:	1 year = 12 months

To begin in a logical way, write the quantity you are given (18 *months*) on the left of an equal sign and the unit you want to change it to (*years*) on the right side, as follows:

$$18 \text{ months} = ? \text{ years}$$

It may help to write 18 *months* as the fraction $\dfrac{18 \text{ months}}{1}$. Thus, you now have:

$$\frac{18 \text{ months}}{1} = ? \text{ years}$$

Develop the appropriate unit fraction

To change *months* to *years*, you need an equivalence between *months* and *years*. That equivalence is:

$$12 \text{ months} = 1 \text{ year}$$

From this equivalence, you can get two possible unit fractions:

$$\frac{12 \text{ months}}{1 \text{ year}} \quad \text{and} \quad \frac{1 \text{ year}}{12 \text{ months}}$$

61

But which of these fractions shall you choose? If you multiply $\dfrac{18 \text{ months}}{1}$ by the first of these fractions, you get:

$$\downarrow \qquad\qquad \downarrow$$

$$\frac{18 \text{ months}}{1} \times \frac{12 \text{ months}}{1 \text{ year}}$$

Notice that both the *months* units are in the numerators of the fractions. Because no cancellation of the units is possible in this case, do not select this unit fraction.

If instead you multiply by the second of the unit fractions, you get the following:

$$\downarrow$$

$$\frac{18 \text{ months}}{1} \times \frac{1 \text{ year}}{12 \text{ months}} = ? \text{ years}$$

$$\uparrow$$

Notice that now *one of the months is in the numerator (top), and the other month is in the denominator (bottom) of a fraction.* Because cancellation of the *months* is now possible, this is the appropriate unit fraction to choose.

Cancel the units of measurement

$$\frac{18 \; \cancel{\text{months}}}{1} \times \frac{1 \text{ year}}{12 \; \cancel{\text{months}}} = ? \text{ years}$$

After you cancel the *months*, notice that *year* (the unit of measurement that you want to find) is the only remaining unit on the left side:

$$\frac{18 \; \cancel{\text{months}}}{1} \times \frac{\boxed{1 \text{ year}}}{12 \; \cancel{\text{months}}} = ? \text{ years}$$

Cancel the numbers and finish the multiplication

After you are sure that you have *only the unit of measurement that you want (years) remaining on the left side and that it is on the top of a fraction,* you can complete the cancellation and multiplication of the numbers as follows:

$$\frac{\overset{3}{\cancel{18}} \; \cancel{\text{months}}}{1} \times \frac{1 \text{ year}}{\underset{2}{\cancel{12}} \; \cancel{\text{months}}} = \frac{3 \text{ years}}{2} \quad \text{or} \quad 1\frac{1}{2} \text{ years}$$

So, 18 *months* is equivalent to $1\frac{1}{2}$ *years*.

> ### Stop and think
>
> To convert one unit to another first identify the unit fraction, simplify the numbers and ensure that the unit (weight/amount, etc.) that you want is on the top of the fraction. Consider monitoring and reporting a patient's daily fluid intake: you may wish to convert millilitres of a liquid into litres.

Example 3.1

Change $2\frac{1}{4}$ *hours* to an equivalent amount of time in *minutes*. The elements in this problem are:

The given quantity: $2\frac{1}{4}$ hours

The quantity you want to find: ? minutes

An equivalence between them: 1 hour = 60 minutes

$$2\frac{1}{4} \text{ hours} = ? \text{ minutes}$$

Avoid doing multiplication with mixed numbers; change them to improper fractions or decimal numbers. In this case, you can write $2\frac{1}{4}$ *hours* as the improper fraction $\frac{9}{4}$ *hours*.

It is better to write the quantity $\frac{9}{4}$ *hours* as $\dfrac{9 \text{ hours}}{4}$ in order to make it clear that the unit

of measurement (*hours*) is in the numerator of the fraction, not in the denominator. So, the problem becomes

$$\frac{9 \text{ hours}}{4} = ? \text{ minutes}$$

Identify the appropriate unit fraction

You want to change *hours* to *minutes*, so you need an equivalence between *hours* and *minutes*. That equivalence is:

$$1 \text{ hour} = 60 \text{ minutes}$$

From this equivalence, you get two possible fractions, which are both equal to 1:

$$\frac{1 \text{ hour}}{60 \text{ minutes}} \quad \text{and} \quad \frac{60 \text{ minutes}}{1 \text{ hour}}$$

But which of these fractions will lead to cancellation? Because you want to eliminate (cancel) the *hours*, and because *hours* are on the top, as follows:

$$\frac{9 \text{ hours}}{4} = ? \text{ minutes}$$

you need to multiply by the unit fraction with *hour* on the bottom, as follows:

$$\frac{9 \text{ hours}}{4} \times \frac{60 \text{ minutes}}{1 \text{ hour}} = ? \text{ minutes}$$

This is what you want because cancellation of the *hour(s)* is now possible.

Cancel the units

$$\frac{9 \ \cancel{\text{hours}}}{4} \times \frac{60 \text{ minutes}}{1 \ \cancel{\text{hour}}} = ? \text{ minutes}$$

After you cancel the *hour(s)*, make sure that *minutes* (the unit you want) is the only remaining unit of measurement and that it is in a numerator (top) of a fraction:

$$\frac{9 \text{ hours}}{4} \times \frac{60 \text{ minutes}}{1 \text{ hour}} = ? \text{ minutes}$$

Cancel the numbers and finish the multiplication

$$\frac{9 \text{ hours}}{\overset{4}{1}} \times \frac{\overset{15}{60} \text{ minutes}}{1 \text{ hour}} = 135 \text{ minutes}$$

So, $2\frac{1}{4}$ hours = <u>135 minutes</u>.

Stop and think

To eliminate a particular unit of measurement in the numerator (top), use a unit fraction with that same unit of measurement in the denominator (bottom). Consider the patient who may need 2 litres of fluid intravenously in 24 hours. You may need to work this out in minutes so that you can ensure the fluid volume is given at a steady rate over the time.

Note

When a unit of measure follows a numerical fraction, write the unit of measure in the numerator (top) of the fraction. For example, write $\frac{1}{2}$ hour, as in other words this means 1 hour divided by 2 because the denominator is the number to divide by!

Example 3.2

Note that whilst we work in metric measurements there are occasions when we or the patient may use imperial measurements such as feet and inches. So, change $5\frac{1}{2}$ feet to an equivalent length in inches.

The given quantity:	$5\frac{1}{2}$ feet
The quantity you want to find:	? inches
An equivalence between them:	1 foot = 12 inches

$$5\frac{1}{2} \text{ feet} = ? \text{ inches}$$

$$\frac{11 \text{ feet}}{2} = ? \text{ inches}$$

You want to cancel *feet* and get the answer in *inches*, so choose a fraction with *feet* (*foot*) on the bottom and *inches* on top. You need a fraction that looks like $\dfrac{?\text{ inches}}{?\text{ foot}}$.

Since 1 foot = 12 inches, therefore the fraction is $\dfrac{12\text{ inches}}{1\text{ foot}}$:

$$\frac{11\text{ feet}}{\cancel{2}} \times \frac{\cancel{12}^{\,6}\text{ inches}}{1\text{ foot}} = 66 \text{ inches}$$

So, $5\frac{1}{2}$ feet = 66 inches.

This process can be applied to a wide variety of problems, for example currency exchange as demonstrated by Example 3.3.

Example 3.3

If the exchange rate in a country is 1.25 Euro (E) for 1 pound sterling (£), how many euro (E) will be exchanged for £45?

The given quantity:	£45
The quantity you want to find:	? euros
An equivalence between them:	1.25 euros = £1
	£45 = ? euros

You want to cancel £ and get the answer in *euros*. So, multiply £45 by a fraction that looks like $\dfrac{?\text{ Euros}}{£?}$. Because 1.25 euros = £1, the fraction you want is $\dfrac{1.25\text{ Euros}}{£1}$. Cancel the £signs and do the multiplication to get:

$$\frac{£45}{1} \times \frac{1.25\text{ Euros}}{£1} = 56.25 \text{ Euros.}$$

So, £45 will be exchanged for 56.25 Euros.

Note that this is approximate as exchange rates vary and also they are almost never whole numbers!

Complex problems with single units of measurement

Sometimes you will encounter problems that will require the steps used previously to be repeated one or more times. We call such problems **complex**. In a complex problem, multiplication by more than one unit fraction is required. The method is very similar to that used with simple problems.

Here is an example: Suppose that you cannot wait to see your favourite television programme and want to count down the time in seconds, but it is not on for four hours!! Therefore you want to change *4 hours* to an equivalent time in *seconds*.

The given quantity: 4 hours

The quantity you want to find: ? seconds

An equivalence between them: ?

Most people do not know the direct equivalence between hours and seconds, but you do know the following two equivalences related to the units of measurement in this problem: 1 hour = 60 minutes and 1 minute = 60 seconds. So the problem is:

$$4 \text{ hours} = ? \text{ seconds}$$

or

$$\frac{4 \text{ hours}}{1} = ? \text{ minutes}$$

First, you want to cancel *hours*. To do this, you must use an equivalence containing *hours* and a unit fraction with *hours* on the bottom. Because 1 hour = 60 minutes, this fraction will be $\dfrac{60 \text{ minutes}}{1 \text{ hour}}$:

$$\frac{4 \cancel{\text{ hours}}}{1} \times \frac{60 \text{ minutes}}{1 \cancel{\text{ hour}}} = ? \text{ seconds}$$

After the *hours* are cancelled, as shown previously, only *minutes* remain on the left side. So, what you have done at this point is changed 4 *hours* to (4 × 60 = 240) *minutes*, but you want to obtain the answer in *seconds*. Therefore, the *minutes* must now be cancelled. Because *minutes* is in the numerator, a fraction with *minutes* in the denominator is required. Because 1 *minute* = 60 *seconds*, the fraction is $\dfrac{60 \text{ seconds}}{1 \text{ minute}}$. Now multiplying by this unit fraction, you get:

$$\frac{4 \cancel{\text{ hours}}}{1} \times \frac{60 \text{ minutes}}{1 \cancel{\text{ hour}}} \times \frac{60 \text{ seconds}}{1 \text{ minute}} = ? \text{ seconds}$$

Cancel the *minutes* and notice that the only unit of measurement remaining on the left side is *seconds*, the unit that you want to find!

$$\frac{4 \cancel{\text{ hours}}}{1} \times \frac{60 \cancel{\text{ minutes}}}{1 \cancel{\text{ hour}}} \times \frac{60 \cancel{\text{ seconds}}}{1 \cancel{\text{ minute}}} = ? \text{ seconds}$$

Now that you have the unit of measurement that you want (seconds) on the left side, cancel the numbers (not possible in this example) and finish the multiplication:

$$\frac{4 \cancel{\text{ hours}}}{1} \times \frac{60 \cancel{\text{ minutes}}}{1 \cancel{\text{ hour}}} \times \frac{60 \text{ seconds}}{1 \cancel{\text{ minute}}} = 14\,400 \text{ seconds}$$

So, 4 *hours* is equivalent to 14 400 *seconds*.

Example 3.4

Convert 50 400 *minutes* to an equivalent time in *days*.

The given quantity:	50 400 minutes
The quantity you want to find:	? days
Equivalences between them:	?

You might not know the direct equivalence between minutes and days, but you do know the following two equivalences related to the units in this problem: 60 minutes = 1 hour and 24 hours = 1 day.

$$50\ 400 \text{ minutes} = ? \text{ days}$$

You want to cancel *minutes*. To do this, you must use an equivalence containing *minutes* and make a unit fraction with *minutes* on the bottom. Since 60 minutes = 1 hour, this fraction will be $\dfrac{1 \text{ hour}}{60 \text{ minutes}}$:

$$50\ 400 \cancel{\text{ minutes}} \times \frac{1 \text{ hour}}{60 \cancel{\text{ minutes}}} = ? \text{ days}$$

After the *minutes* are cancelled as shown above, only *hour* remains on the left side, but you want to obtain the answer in *days*. Therefore, the *hour* must now be cancelled. This will require a unit fraction with *hours* in the denominator. Because 1 day = 24 hours, this fraction is $\dfrac{1 \text{ day}}{24 \text{ hours}}$. After cancelling the *hours*, you now have:

$$50\ 400 \cancel{\text{ minutes}} \times \frac{1 \cancel{\text{ hour}}}{60 \cancel{\text{ minutes}}} \times \frac{1 \text{ (day)}}{24 \cancel{\text{ hours}}} = ? \text{ days}$$

Because only *day* (in the numerator) is on the left side, the numbers can be cancelled:

$$\overset{840}{\cancel{50\ 400}} \cancel{\text{ minutes}} \times \frac{1 \cancel{\text{ hour}}}{\underset{1}{\cancel{60}} \cancel{\text{ minutes}}} \times \frac{1 \text{ day}}{24 \cancel{\text{ hours}}} = \frac{840}{24} \text{ days} = 35 \text{ days}$$

So, 50 400 minutes = 35 days. As you could ignore the 1s in the numerators you could simply divide 50 400 by 60 and then divide again by 24.

Note

To make the problem simpler, you do not have to always write 50 400 *minutes* as the fraction $\dfrac{50\ 400 \text{ minutes}}{1}$. If you do this, however, remember that the quantity, 50 400 *minutes*, is understood to be in the numerator of a fraction. Therefore, the 50 400 *minutes* can be divided or cancelled only with a quantity in the denominator of another fraction.

Example 3.5

Kim is having a barbeque for 24 people and is serving beefburgers. Each person will eat 2 beefburgers. How much will the beefburgers for the barbeque cost if a packet of 8 beefburgers costs £2.50?

The given single unit of measurement: 24 people or 24 persons

The single unit of measurement you want to find: ? Cost (£)

You might not know the direct relationship or equivalence between people and cost. But you do know the following equivalents supplied in this problem:

2 beefburgers per person   2 beefburgers = 1 person

1 packet of beefburgers is £2.50   1 packet = £2.50

1 packet has 8 beefburgers   1 packet = 8 beefburgers

But where do you start?

In this problem, there are two single units of measurement—one that is given (persons) and one you have to find (cost). Cost involves a single unit of measurement, namely pounds sterling (£). *Because you are looking for a quantity measured in a single unit of measurement (£), you should start with the given single unit of measurement* (persons):

$$24 \text{ persons} = ? \text{ £}$$

You want to cancel *persons*. To do this, you must use an equivalence containing *person(s)* to make a fraction with *person(s)* on the bottom. From the preceding equivalence, 2 beefburgers = 1 person, this fraction will be $\dfrac{2 \text{ beefburgers}}{\text{person}}$:

$$24 \cancel{\text{ persons}} \times \frac{2 \text{ beefburgers}}{\cancel{\text{person}}} = ?£$$

After the *person(s)* are cancelled, only *beefburgers* remains on the left side, and it indicates that 48 *beefburgers* are needed. But you want to obtain the answer in £. Therefore, the *beefburgers* must now be cancelled. This will require a fraction with *beefburgers* in the denominator. From the equivalence 1 packet = 8 beefburgers, the unit fraction is $\dfrac{1 \text{ packet}}{8 \text{ beefburgers}}$. Thus, you now have:

$$24 \cancel{\text{ persons}} \times \frac{2 \cancel{\text{ beefburgers}}}{\cancel{\text{person}}} \times \frac{1 \text{ packet}}{8 \cancel{\text{ beefburgers}}} = ?£$$

After the *beefburgers* are cancelled, only *packet* remains on the left side, and (if you do the mathematics now) it indicates the number of *packets* (6) that are needed. But you want to obtain the answer in £. Therefore, the *packet* must now be cancelled. This will require a fraction with *packet* in the denominator. From the equivalence 1 packet = £2.50, the unit fraction is $\dfrac{£2.50}{1 \text{ packet}}$:

$$24 \; \overline{\text{persons}} \times \frac{2 \; \overline{\text{beefburgers}}}{\overline{\text{person}}} \times \frac{1 \; \overline{\text{packet}}}{8 \; \overline{\text{beefburgers}}} \times \frac{\text{£}2.50}{1 \; \overline{\text{packet}}} = ? \text{£}$$

Because you now have only £ (in the numerator) on the left side, the numbers can be cancelled and the multiplication finished:

$$\overset{3}{\cancel{24}} \; \overline{\text{persons}} \times \frac{2 \; \overline{\text{beefburgers}}}{\overline{\text{person}}} \times \frac{1 \; \overline{\text{packet}}}{8 \; \overline{\text{beefburgers}}} \times \frac{\text{£}2.50}{1 \; \overline{\text{packet}}} = \text{£}15$$

So, the beefburgers for the party will cost £15.00.

Note

Don't stop multiplying by unit fractions until the unit of measurement you are looking for is the only remaining unit on the left side. Remember that the unit you are looking for must end up in the numerator of a fraction (top). The example given could just as easily be costing a daily meal replacement drink for a patient or identifying how much stock of a particular medication you would need to order to cover a public holiday period.

Changing one rate to another rate

A rate is a fraction with different units of measurement on top compared with on the bottom. For example, 50 *miles* per *hour* written as 50 miles/hour and 3 *pounds* per *week* written as 3 pounds/week are rates. In a dosage calculation, the bottom unit of measurement is frequently time (for example, *hours* or *minutes*). We sometimes want to change one rate into another rate. These problems are done in a manner similar to the method that was used to do the single-unit-to-single-unit problems.

Simple problems with rates

Example 3.6

Convert *5 metres per hour* to an equivalent rate of speed in *centimetres per hour*.

The given rate: 5 metres per hour

The rate you want to find: ? centimetres per hour

Because you are looking for a *rate*, you start with the **given rate**:

5 metres per hour = ? centimetres per hour

Write these rates as fractions:

$$\frac{5 \; \text{metres}}{\text{hour}} = \frac{\text{centimetres}}{\text{hour}}$$

Notice that you are given a rate with *hour* in the denominator, and the rate you are looking for also has *hour* in the denominator. Therefore, *the denominator does not have to be changed!*

But the given rate has metres in the numerator, and the rate you want has a different unit, *centimetres*, in the numerator. Therefore, *metres* must be changed. To cancel *metres*, you must use an equivalence containing *metres*, namely, 100 cm = 1 *metre*. Because metres is in the numerator, you need a unit fraction with metres in the denominator. This unit fraction is $\dfrac{100\ cm}{1m}$. After the *metres* are cancelled, centimetres remain on top, and *hour* remains on the bottom, and those are the units you want. Finally, do the multiplication of the numbers:

$$\frac{5\ \cancel{m}}{\cancel{hour}} \times \frac{100\ \cancel{cm}}{1\ \cancel{m}} = \frac{500\ cm}{1\ hour}$$

So, 5 *metres per hour* is equivalent to 500 *centimetres per hour*.

Example 3.7

Convert 90 *centimetres per hour* to an equivalent rate in *centimetres per minute*.

The given rate: 90 cm/h

The rate you want to find: ? cm/min

Since you are looking for a rate, you start with the given rate:

$$90\ cm\ per\ hour = ?\ cm\ per\ minute$$

Write these rates as fractions:

$$\frac{90\ cm}{h} = \frac{?\ cm}{min}$$

Notice that you are given a rate with *cm* in the numerator, and the answer you are looking for also has *cm* in the numerator. Therefore, the numerator does not have to be changed!

But the given rate has *h* in the denominator, and the rate you want has a different unit, *min*, in the denominator. Therefore, *h* must be eliminated. Since *h* is in the denominator, you need a fraction with *h* in the numerator. Use the equivalence 1 h = 60 min. This unit fraction is $\dfrac{1\ h}{60\ min}$:

$$\frac{90\ \cancel{cm}}{\cancel{h}} \times \frac{1\ \cancel{h}}{60\ \cancel{min}} = \frac{?\ cm}{min}$$

After the *h* is cancelled, *cm* remains on top and *min* is on the bottom, and those are the units you want. Cancel the numbers and finish the multiplication:

$$\frac{\overset{3}{\cancel{90}}\ cm}{\cancel{h}} \times \frac{1\ \cancel{h}}{\underset{2}{\cancel{60}}\ min} = \frac{3\ cm}{2\ min} = \frac{1.5\ cm}{min}$$

So, 90 *cm/hour* is equivalent to a rate of 1.5 *cm/minute*.

Practice point

Rates are apparent all the time in healthcare and nursing, e.g. peak flow readings can be recorded as L/min or ml/sec, you may monitor urine output as ml/hour or ml/min, etc. Not all require changing but some might so it is useful to know how to do this for reasons other than drug administration.

Complex problems with rates

Example 3.8

Convert $10\frac{1}{2}$ *metres/hour* to an equivalent rate in *centimetres/minute*.

The given rate: $10\frac{1}{2}$ metres/hour

The rate you want to find: ? centimetres/minute

Since you are looking for a rate, you should start with a rate:

$$10\frac{1}{2} \text{ metres/hour} = ? \text{ centimetres/minute}$$

Write $10\frac{1}{2}$ as the improper fraction $\frac{21}{2}$:

$$\frac{21 \text{ cm}}{2 \text{ h}} = \frac{? \text{ cm}}{\text{min}}$$

You want to cancel m. To do this, you must use an equivalence containing m on the bottom. Because you want to convert to *centimetres*, use the equivalence 100 cm = 1 metre, and the unit fraction will be $\dfrac{100 \text{ cm}}{1 \text{ m}}$:

$$\frac{21 \text{ m}}{2 \text{ h}} \times \frac{100 \text{ cm}}{1 \text{ m}} = \frac{? \text{ cm}}{\text{min}}$$

After the m is cancelled, cm is on top, which is what you want. But h is on the bottom and it must be cancelled. This will require a fraction with h in the numerator. From the equivalence 1 hour = 60 minutes, the unit fraction is $\dfrac{1 \text{ h}}{60 \text{ min}}$. After cancelling the hours, you now have:

$$\frac{21 \text{ m}}{2 \text{ h}} \times \frac{100 \text{ cm}}{1 \text{ m}} \times \frac{1 \text{ h}}{60 \text{ min}} = \frac{? \text{ cm}}{\text{min}}$$

You now have *in* on top and *min* on the bottom, so do the cancelling and multiplications of the numbers.

$$\frac{21 \text{ m}}{2 \text{ h}} \times \frac{100 \text{ cm}}{1 \text{ m}} \times \frac{1 \text{ h}}{60 \text{ min}} = \frac{17.5 \text{ cm}}{\text{min}}$$

So, $10\frac{1}{2}$ m/hour = 17.5 cm/minute.

> ### Stop and think
>
> Writing out problems will help to see how measurements relate to each other. Do not rely on mental arithmetic for every problem. In nursing there are often complex problems which may need working out, such as converting litres/hour to mls/min or even giving drugs based on body weight mg/kg/day. An asthmatic patient is advised to record their peak expiratory flow (PEF) rate daily. If their PEF rate falls below 300 L/min the patient will need to seek urgent assistance, however, the reading the patient reports is 60 ml/sec which seems low. You look further and on calculation find this equates to 360 L/min – the advice is to record the PEF in the same units regularly, but you realise you can convert the readings if you need to.

Summary

In this chapter, the techniques of conversion from one measurement to another was introduced.

The following mathematical concepts were reinforced

+ A nonzero number divided by itself equals 1.
+ A fraction equal to 1 is called a unit fraction.
+ When a quantity is multiplied (or divided) by 1, the quantity is unchanged.
+ Cancellation always involves a quantity in a numerator and another quantity in a denominator.

Simple single-unit-to-single-unit problems

+ Start with the **given** single unit of measure on the left side of the = sign.
+ Write the single unit of measure you want to **find** on the right side of the = sign.
+ Identify an **equivalence** containing the units of measure in the problem.
+ Use the equivalence to make a unit fraction with the **given** unit of measure in the **denominator**.
+ Multiply by the unit fraction.
+ Cancel the units of measure. The only unit of measurement remaining on the left side (in a numerator) will match the unit of measure on the right side.
+ Cancel the numbers and finish the multiplication.

Simple rate-to-rate problems

+ Start with the **given** rate on the left side of the equal sign.
+ Write the rate you want to **find** on the right side of the equal sign.
+ Identify a unit of measure that must be cancelled.

+ Find an **equivalence** containing the unwanted unit of measure you want to cancel.

+ Choose a unit fraction that leads to cancellation of the unwanted unit of measurement.

+ Cancel the units of measurement. The only units of measurement remaining on the left side (in a numerator) will match the units of measure on the right side.

+ Cancel the numbers and finish the multiplication.

+ In medical dosage calculations involving rates of flow, time (in minutes or hours) will always be in the denominator.

Complex problems

+ Repeat the preceding steps until the only unit of measurement(s) remaining on the left side is the same as the unit of measurement(s) on the right side.

Practice sets

The answers to *Try these for practice* and *Exercises* appear in Appendix A at the end of the book.

Try these for practice

Test your comprehension after reading the chapter.

1. How many minutes are in 4.5 hours? _____

2. An infant weighs 7 lb 3 oz. What is this weight in ounces? _____

3. How many hours are in $1\frac{1}{2}$ weeks? _____

4. Water is flowing from a hose at 100 mL per minute. Find this rate of flow in litres per hour. _____

5. A certain animal eats 250 gs of food per day. At this rate, find the number of *kilograms of food per week* the animal eats. _____

Exercises

Reinforce your understanding in class or at home.

1. 1.5 min = _____ sec

2. $5\frac{1}{2}$ yr = _____ mon

3. $4\frac{1}{2}$ day = _____ h

4. $\dfrac{3}{4}$ h = _____ min

5. 51 mon = _____ yr

6. 3 L = _____ mL

7. 3 kg = _____ g

8. $\dfrac{100 \text{ cm}}{\text{sec}} = \dfrac{\text{____}\ m}{\text{sec}}$

9. $\dfrac{30 \text{ L}}{\text{min}} = \dfrac{\text{____}\ L}{\text{sec}}$

10. $\dfrac{60 \text{ km}}{\text{h}} = \dfrac{\text{____}\ m}{\text{min}}$

11. What fraction of an hour is 2700 seconds? _____

12. Change 1680 hours to weeks. _____

13. Write 1 209 600 seconds as an equivalent amount of time in weeks. _____

14. There are 24 cans of soft drink in a case. Each can contains 330 mL. Every 100 mL of soft drink contains 10 g of sugar. How many kilograms of sugar are in 5 cases of soft drink? _____

Chapter 4

The metric measurement system

Learning outcomes

After completing this chapter, you will be able to

1. Identify the units of measurement in the metric system.

2. Recognise the abbreviations for the units of measurement.

3. State the equivalents for the units of volume for liquids.

4. State the equivalents for the units of weight for solids.

5. Convert from one unit to another within the metric three system.

The *International System (SI)*, commonly known as the *metric system*, is replacing other imperial systems of measurement. However, other systems are still in use, and in a more prevalent manner than in the United Kingdom (UK), especially in countries such as the United States of America (USA). You should appreciate their existence whilst also understanding that in Europe the SI system of measurement ensures comparability across countries and literature. There are plenty of examples of use of imperial measures in the UK (i.e. distance is measured in miles), but for medication and weights and measures in general the metric system is preferred whilst for trade and business use of the metric system is mandatory and monitored by law (NWML 2008). The metric system uses whole and decimal numbers (i.e. 3.5); at times fractions (i.e. $3\frac{1}{2}$) may be utilised. The purpose of this chapter is to explore and clarify metric measurements and to develop confidence in using and moving between decimals and fractions.

Diagnostic questions

Before commencing this chapter try the following questions to stimulate your appetite. Compare your answers with those in Appendix A.

1. Which is larger 5.17 or 5.38?

2. Which is smaller 2.19 or 2.64?

3. Put these in size order, the largest first:

    75.1   25.7   25.762   0.34   3.44

4. Put these in order, the smallest first:

    0.96   0.547   0.009   1.76   0.19

5. Write three and four tenths as a decimal using digits.

The metric system

The metric system is the most widely used, general system of measurement in the world and is the preferred system for prescribing medications. The fundamental units of measurement in the metric system are the **litre** (for liquid volume), the **gram** (for weight) and the **metre** (for length). Other units are formed by placing prefixes onto these fundamental units. The prefixes commonly used in medical doses are **kilo**, **centi**, **milli** and **micro**. The equivalences illustrated in this section need to be understood in order to work within the metric system.

> **Note**
>
> The abbreviation **mL** should be used instead of the abbreviation cc because 'c' may be confused with 'u' (units) or 'cc' with '00' (double zero). Whilst 'cc' is not generally used for medicine measures it is seen occasionally in relation to volumes and may well be seen in international texts.

Liquid volume measurements

Drugs in liquid form are measured by volume. The volume of a liquid is the amount of space it occupies. In dosage calculations, *litres* and *millilitres* are used to measure liquid volume (see Table 4.1).

Table 4.1 Metric equivalents of liquid volume

1 litre (L) = 1000 millilitres (mL)
1000 microlitres = 1 millilitre (mL)

Originally, units for volume and mass were directly related to each other, with mass defined in terms of a volume of water. Even though that definition is no longer used, the relation is quite close at room temperature. So as a practical matter, one can fill a container with water and weigh it to get the volume. For example:

1000 litres	= 1 cubic metre	≈ 1 tonne of water
1 litre	= 1 cubic decimetre	≈ 1 kilogram of water
1 millilitre	= 1 cubic centimetre	≈ 1 gram of water
1 microlitre	= 1 cubic millimetre	≈ 1 milligram of water

Millilitres are used for smaller amounts of fluids. The prefix milli means $\frac{1}{1000}$, so:

$$1 \text{ litre (L)} = 1000 \text{ millilitres (mL)}$$

Millilitres are equivalent to *cubic centimetres* (cm^3 or cc), so:

$$1 \text{ mL} = 1 \text{ cm}^3 = 1 \text{ cc}$$

Note: This (cc) term is not generally used in the United Kingdom or Europe but, due to the prevalence of American texts and electronic resources, it is always useful to understand the equivalences.

It is straightforward to convert fractions to decimals. The unit fraction has the *given units of measurement on the bottom* (the denominator) and the *desired units of measurement on top* (the numerator), you simply divide the top number by the bottom number, as the following examples show.

Example 4.1

If a patient is prescribed 0.5 L of 5% glucose in water, how many millilitres were ordered?

$$0.5 \text{ L} = ? \text{ mL}$$

Cancel the litres and obtain the equivalent amount in millilitres:

$$0.5 \text{ L} \times \frac{? \text{ mL}}{? \text{ L}} = ? \text{ mL}$$

Because 1000 mL = 1 L, the fraction you want is $\dfrac{1000 \text{ mL}}{1 \text{ L}}$:

$$0.5 \text{ L} \times \frac{1000 \text{ mL}}{1 \text{ L}} = 500 \text{ mL}$$

So, the patient is prescribed <u>500 mL</u> of 5% glucose in water.

Stop and think

When reporting or writing volumes such as 0.5 L this is best written as decimals instead of $\frac{5}{10}$ or $\frac{1}{2}$ L in the metric system to avoid confusion.

Practice point

When using decimal points the zero needs to be used in numbers less than 1 (e.g. 0.5). When used with whole numbers above 1 this can cause confusion. For example, 3.0 could be confused as 30 or .1 can be confused as 1. Be cautious with the use of zeros and decimal points – a dose of 2.0 mg of a drug maybe confused for 20 mg of a drug and potentially causes serious harm to a patient.

Example 4.2

Your patient is to receive *1750 mL of 0.9% sodium chloride (NaCl intravenously (IV)) every 12 hours*. What is the same amount in litres?

$$1750 \text{ mL} = ? \text{ L}$$

Cancel the millilitres and obtain the equivalent amount in litres.

$$1750 \text{ mL} \times \frac{? \text{ L}}{? \text{ mL}} = ? \text{ L}$$

Because 1000 mL = 1 L, the fraction you want is $\dfrac{1 \text{ L}}{1000 \text{ mL}}$

$$1750 \text{ mL} \times \frac{1 \text{ L}}{1000 \text{ mL}} = \frac{1750 \text{ L}}{1000} = 1.75 \text{ L}$$

So, 1750 mL of 0.9% NaCl is the same amount as <u>1.75 L</u> of 0.9% NaCl.

Alert

The abbreviation for microgram, mcg, is preferred over the abbreviation μg because μg may be mistaken for the abbreviation for milligram, mg. This error would result in a dose that would be 1000 times greater than the prescribed dose – the heart medication digoxin could be prescribed as 62.5 μg or 0.0625 mg, thus giving 62.5 mg would be 1000 times too much and extremely serious for the patient.

Weight measures

Drugs in dry form are measured by weight in the metric system. In dosage calculations, **kilograms**, **grams**, **milligrams** and **micrograms** (written in order of size) are used to measure weight. *Kilograms* are the largest of these units of measurement and *micrograms* are the smallest (see Table 4.2).

Table 4.2 Metric equivalents of weight

1 kilogram (kg) = 1000 grams (g)
1 gram (g) = 1000 milligrams (mg)
1 milligram (mg) = 1000 micrograms (mcg)

Kilograms are used for heavier weights. The prefix kilo means 1000, so:

$$1 \textbf{ kilo} \text{gram (kg)} = 1000 \textit{ grams} \text{ (g)}$$

Milligrams are used for lighter weights, and *micrograms* are used for even lighter weights. The prefix milli means $\dfrac{1}{1000}$, and micro means $\dfrac{1}{1\,000\,000}$, so:

1 gram (g) = 1000 **milli**grams (mg)

1 milligram (mg) = 1000 **micro**grams (mcg or μg)

Using the simple conversion information in Table 4.2, you can convert a quantity written in one unit of metric weight to an equivalent quantity in another unit of metric weight. The following examples show you how to do this.

Example 4.3

The prescription states *125 mcg of Lanoxin (digoxin) PO daily*. How many milligrams of this cardiac medication would you administer to the patient?

$$125 \text{ mcg} = ? \text{ mg}$$

Cancel the micrograms and obtain the equivalent amount in milligrams:

$$125 \text{ mcg} \times \frac{? \text{ mg}}{? \text{ mcg}} = ? \text{ mg}$$

Because 1000 mcg = 1 mg, you have

$$125 \text{ mcg} \times \frac{1 \text{ mg}}{1000 \text{ mcg}} = 0.125 \text{ mg}$$

So, 125 mcg is the same amount as 0.125 mg, and you would administer 0.125 mg of digoxin.

Example 4.4

The prescription states *Glipizide 15 mg PO daily before breakfast*. How many grams of this hypoglycaemic agent would you administer?

$$15 \text{ mg} = ? \text{ g}$$

Cancel the milligrams and obtain the equivalent amount in grams:

$$15 \text{ mg} \times \frac{? \text{ g}}{? \text{ mg}} = ? \text{ g}$$

$$15 \text{ mg} \times \frac{1 \text{ g}}{1000 \text{ mg}} = \frac{15}{1000} \text{ g} = 0.015 \text{ g}$$

So, 15 mg is the same amount as 0.015 g, and you would administer 0.015 g.

Stop and think

Be aware of the relationship between grams (g), milligrams (mg) and micrograms (mcg). Mistaking 62.5 mcg for 62.5 mg means an overdose of 1000 times the prescribed dose! (Because 62.5 mcg = 0.0625 mg)

Length measures

Centimetres (cm) are used to measure lengths or heights and the centimetre (cm) is the only metric unit of length used in medical dosage calculations. Therefore, no conversions of metric units of length are necessary in medical dosage calculations. You may see metres (m) being used, but this would be for non-drug but related aspects, e.g. height or to calculate body mass index. There are 100 centimetres (cm) in a metre (m) so a person who is 1.8 m tall is also 180 cm tall.

Shortcut for converting units in the metric system

The following chart is useful for a quick method of converting units of measurement within the metric system.

	Kilo-	Fundamental unit	Milli-	Micro-
Weight	kilogram (kg)	gram (g)	milligram (mg)	microgram (mcg)
Volume		litre (L)	millilitre (mL)	

Another way of looking at it:

1	Gram/Litre
10	Decigram/litres (not generally used in practice)
100	Centigrams/litres (not generally used in practice)
1 000	**Milligrams/litres**
10 000	**Micrograms/litres**
100 000	**Nanograms/litres**

The metric system, like our number system, is a **decimal** system *because it is based on the number 10*. Therefore, measurements given in one metric unit can be converted to another metric unit by *merely moving the decimal place*. Using the preceding chart indicating the fundamental units and equivalencies, to change a quantity measured in units from one column to units in the column to its right, move the decimal point *three places* to the right. To change a quantity measured in units from one column to units in the column to its left, move the decimal point *three places* to the left. In other words, to make a number bigger (even though the amount is smaller) move the decimal point to the right and to make it smaller move the decimal point to the left. Therefore, Examples 4.1 to 4.4 could also have been done this way as shown in the following examples.

Stop and think

When converting 0.5 L to 500 mL, the unit of measurement got smaller (L to mL), whereas the number got larger (0.5 to 500).

Example 4.5

(Shortcut method) 0.5 L = ? mL

In this problem, you convert from L to mL. The movement from L to mL in the following chart is a movement of one column to the right. Therefore, the conversion is accomplished by moving the decimal point three places to the right.

Kilo-	Fundamental unit	Milli-	Micro-
	litre (L)	millilitre (mL)	

So, 0.5 L = 0 . 5 0 0 mL = 0500. mL = <u>500 mL</u>.

Stop and think

Recall from before – when converting 1750 mL to 1.75 L, the unit of measurement got larger (mL to L), whereas the number got smaller.

Example 4.6

(Shortcut method) 1750 mL = ? L

In this problem, you convert from mL to L. The movement from mL to L in the following chart is a movement of one column to the left. Therefore, the conversion is accomplished by moving the decimal point three places to the left.

Kilo-	Fundamental unit	Milli-	Micro-
	litre (L)	millilitre (mL)	

So, 1750 mL = 1 7 5 0 . L = 1.750 L = <u>1.75 L</u>.

Example 4.7

(Shortcut method) 125 mcg = ? mg

In this problem, you convert from mcg to mg. The movement from mcg to mg in the following chart is a movement of one column to the left. Therefore, the conversion is accomplished by moving the decimal point three places to the left.

Kilo-	Fundamental unit	Milli-	Micro-
Kilogram (kg)	gram (g)	milligram (mg)	microgram (mcg)

So, 125 mcg = 1 2 5. mg = .125 mg = <u>0.125 mg</u>.

Practice point

Because the volume of ordinary household spoons, cups and glasses may vary, medications should *not* be administered using ordinary household utensils. Thus if a patient is prescribed 5 mL of a medicine this should be measured using a specific 5 mL medicine spoon and not a household teaspoon.

Example 4.8

(Shortcut method) 15 mg = ? g

In this problem, you convert from mg to g. The movement from mg to g in the following chart is a movement of one column to the left. Therefore, the conversion is accomplished by moving the decimal point three places to the left.

Kilo-	Fundamental unit	Milli-	Micro-
Kilogram (kg)	gram (g)	milligram (mg)	microgram (mcg)

So, 15 mg = 0 1 5. g = .015 g = <u>0.015 g</u>.

Note

Grams are metric units so they are expressed as decimals or whole numbers. Therefore, $\frac{1}{2}$ gram is expressed as 0.5 gram. In prescribing it is best practice to NOT write amounts less than one in a unit but to change the unit so for amounts less than 1 gram it should be written 500 mg rather than 0.5 g – this will help to eliminate confusion (Smith 2004).

Measurements in the imperial measurement system

The only units of weight used in the imperial system are: ounces (oz), pounds (lb) and stones; although use of these is not actively encouraged, they do exist within clinical situations from time to time. Thus a background knowledge of them is beneficial – it is best not to mix imperial and metric measurements, i.e. weight in stones and height in metres, as this is confusing and also makes calculations such as for Body Mass Index rather difficult. You are advised to adhere to metric units and, if a situation arises where imperial measurements occur, you can make some sense of them. It is also useful to be able to convert weight from pounds and stones to kilograms or grams if the need arises, such as giving advice on body weight to a patient using the equivalences which can act as conversion factors in Table 4.3.

Table 4.3 Weight in the imperial measurement system

16 ounces (oz) = 1 pound (lb)
14 pounds (lbs) = 1 stone
1 ounce (oz) = 28.34 g
1 g = 0.002205 lb
1 lb = 453.59 g

To convert pounds to grams

Multiply the number of pounds you need to measure by the conversion factor identified above to get the equivalent number of grams (pounds × 453.59 = grams).

Example: 3.3 pounds × 453.59 = 1497 grams.

To convert grams to pounds

Multiply the number of grams you need to measure by the conversion factor to get the equivalent number of pounds (grams × 0.0022 = pounds).

Example: 1200 grams × 0.0022 = 2.64 pounds

Stop and think

You may remember using bags of sugar as examples: 1 kg = 2.2 lbs (the same conversion factor as above so: 1000 g × 0.0022 = 2.2 lbs).

Example 4.9

An infant weighs 5 lb 8 oz. What is the weight of the infant in grams and kilograms?

First make the measures the same rather than a mix of lbs and oz. As there are 16 oz in 1 lb, this is converted in steps:

Convert the infant's weight to ounces. First change the 5 lb to ounces:

$$5 \text{ lb} = ? \text{ oz}$$

Cancel the pounds and obtain the equivalent amount in ounces:

$$5 \text{ lb} = \frac{? \text{ oz}}{? \text{ lb}} = ? \text{ oz}$$

Because 16 oz = 1 lb, the fraction is $\dfrac{16 \text{ oz}}{? \text{ lb}}$:

$$5 \cancel{\text{ lb}} \times \frac{16 \, \textcircled{\text{oz}}}{1 \cancel{\text{ lb}}} = 80 \text{ oz}$$

Now add the extra 8 oz.

$$80 \text{ oz} + 8 \text{ oz} = 88 \text{ oz}$$

So, the 5 lb 8 oz infant weighs 88 oz.

Then use the conversion factor to determine the weight in grams:

$$88 \text{ oz} \times 28.34 \text{ g} = \underline{2493.92}$$

$$2493.92 \text{ g} = \underline{2.49 \text{ kg}}$$

Remember to work to a final answer to 2 decimal places.

Because heights are often given in feet and inches, it is useful to be able to convert to centimeters (see Table 4.4 and Example 4.10). Equivalent values for liquid volumes are given in Table 4.5.

Table 4.4 Equivalent values for units of length

Metric	Imperial
2.54 centimetres (cm) = 1 inch (in)	
1 cm = 0.39 in	

To convert inches to centimetres
Multiply the number of inches you have by the conversion factor to get the equivalent number of centimetres (inches × 2.54 = centimetres).

To convert centimetres to inches
Multiply the number of centimetres you have by the conversion factor to get the equivalent number of inches (centimetres × 0.39 = inches).

Table 4.5 Equivalent values for liquid volumes

Metric	Imperial
454 mL =	1 pint
1 L =	$1^{3}/_{4}$ pints

Example 4.10

Adam is 6 feet 3 inches tall. What is his height in centimetres?

$$6 \text{ ft } 3 \text{ in} \quad \text{means} \quad 6 \text{ ft} + 3 \text{ in}$$

First determine Adam's height in inches. To do this, convert 6 ft to inches:

$$6 \text{ ft} = ? \text{ in}$$

You want to cancel feet and obtain the equivalent height in inches:

$$6 \text{ ft} \times \frac{? \text{ in}}{? \text{ ft}} = ? \text{ in}$$

Because 1 ft = 12 in, the fraction is $\dfrac{12 \text{ in}}{1 \text{ ft}}$:

$$6 \text{ ft} \times \frac{12 \text{ in}}{1 \text{ ft}} = 72 \text{ in}$$

Now, add the extra 3 in:

$$72 \text{ in} + 3 \text{ in} = 75 \text{ in}$$

Now convert 75 in to centimetres:

$$75 \text{ in} = ? \text{ cm}$$

You want to cancel inches and obtain the equivalent length in centimetres:

$$75 \text{ in} \times \frac{? \text{ cm}}{? \text{ in}} = ? \text{ cm}$$

Because 1 in = 2.54 cm, thus the fraction is $\dfrac{2.54 \text{ cm}}{1 \text{ in}}$:

$$75 \text{ in} \times \frac{2.54 \text{ cm}}{1 \text{ in}} = 190.5 \text{ cm}$$

So, Adam is 190.5 cm tall.

Stop and think

A short rhyme from school days may assist in remembering volumes:

A litre of water's a pint and three quarters.

Practice points

Medications, which are given but incorrectly identified as milligrams or micrograms, can have serious consequences. Giving a dose of morphine (opiate analgesia) as an incorrect dose – 100 milligrams instead of 10 milligrams – can be serious. Another medication which is often confused is digoxin as medications may be dispensed in milligrams and the prescription is written in micrograms. Thus if a patient is pre-scribed 125 mcg but is given 1.25 mg this can lead to serious heart problem as it should have been 0.125 mg. Further examples can be seen in the Department of Health report on improving medication safety (Smith 2004). It is best to think – does this look like a lot of tablets? Have I got the units of measurements correct? What is the normal dose?

Summary

In this chapter, the metric system of measurement used in medication administration was explored and simple conversion calculations were used to convert between different units within the metric system.

+ The metric system is the principal system and is used uniformly across Europe.
+ Avoid the use of confusing abbreviations (u or µg.)
+ The metric system uses decimal numbers, not fractions.
+ A memorable shortcut method of conversion within the metric system is by moving the decimal point to right or left.

References

National Weights and Measures Laboratory (NWML) (2008) *Legal weights and measures*. Teddington: National Weights and Measures Laboratory. Available at: www.nwml.org.gov/contents.aspx?SCID=257 (accessed March 2009).

Smith J (2004) *Building a Safer NHS for Patients: Improving Medication Safety*. London: HMSO.

Reflection

Consider your daily life – how frequently do measurements appear. Perhaps calorie counting, obtaining discounts in shops or checking your bank balance or paying bills or even comparing prices at petrol stations looking for a good deal? List them here:

_____

_____

What types of measurements appear and what types of calculations do you perform?

_____

_____

Rate your skill in these aspects?

Really poor = 1............2...............3................4................5 = Excellent

Now, consider situations when you use calculations at work, think of all aspects in which they occur (excluding drug calculations). List them:

_____

_____

How do you rate your skill in these?

Really poor = 1............2...............3................4................5 = Excellent

If you feel these aspects are not as good as you wish try the exercises presented and then reassess yourself. Try to look in your cupboards at home and identify weights and measures – even whilst shopping – try to convert grams to milligrams or litres to millilitres or even imperial to metric measures (pints to litres) to give you further practice.

Practice sets

The answers to *Try these for practice*, *Exercises* and *Cumulative review exercises* appear in Appendix A at the end of the book.

Try these for practice

Test your comprehension after reading the chapter.

1. Fill in the missing numbers in the following chart.

(a) 1 L   = _____ mL

(b) 10 L   = _____ mL

(c) 1 kg   = _____ g

(d) 1 g   = _____ mg

(e) 1 mg   = _____ mcg

(f) 10 mg = _____ mcg

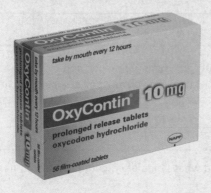

Figure 4.1 Product carton for
Oxycontin® tablets

(Reprinted with the permission of Napp
Pharmaceuticals Limited)

2. Use the carton in Figure 4.1 to determine the number of grams of oxycodone in 1 tablet
of the drug.

3. The prescriber prescribes *methorexate 2.5 mg PO BD*, for a patient with psoriasis. How
many micrograms of this drug are administered in a day?

4. The urinary output of a patient with an indwelling Foley catheter is 1800 mL. How many
litres of urine are in the bag?

5. If a patient drank $1\frac{1}{2}$ litres of water, how many millitres of water did the patient drink?

Exercises

Reinforce your understanding in class or at home.

1. 400 mg = _____ g

2. 0.003 g = _____ mg

3. 0.07 g   = _____ mg

4. 3 L   = _____ mL

5. 2500 mL = _____ L

6. 600 mcg = _____ mg

7. Using the drug label in Figure 4.2, determine the number of micrograms of valsartan
(Diovan) in one tablet.

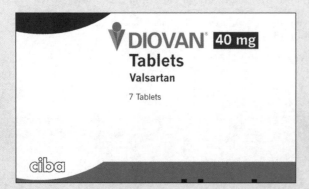

Figure 4.2 Drug label for Diovan

(Reproduced with permission of Novartis
Pharmaceuticals Ltd. Sample. For educational
use only.)

PHARMACY STAMP:	AGE: 78	NAME (INCLUDING FORENAME) AND ADDRESS: *Abdul Danuish* *2 Otter Lane* *Big Town BG 234 9BG*		
	D.O.B 24/12/30	NHS NUMBER: *AD 1234*		
DISPENSER'S ENDORSEMENT	NUMBER OF DAYS TREATMENT. N.B ENSURE DOSE IS STATED		NP	PRICING OFFICE
PACK & QUANTITY	*Chlorpromazine 50 mg PO three times a day (8 hourly) for three (3) days*			
SIGNATURE OF DOCTORS *R. Green*			DATE: *19/04/09*	
FOR DISPENSER NO. OF ITEMS ON FORM	DOCTOR ADDRESS AND TELEPHONE NUMBER: *R. Green* *Anytown High Street Surgery* *High Street* *Old Town WD9 7GB*			
PLEASE READ NOTES OVERLEAF				

Figure 4.3 Drug prescription sheet

8. A patient is to have a loading dose of *digoxin 520 mcg PO stat*. How many milligrams are in this dose?

9. According to the prescripton sheet in Figure 4.3, what is the dose in grams of the chlorpromazine?

10. A patient is drinking $\frac{1}{2}$ litre of orange juice every 2 hours. At this rate, how many millilitres of orange juice will the patient drink in 8 hours?

11. An infant weighs 3400 grams. How much does the infant weigh in kilograms?

12. A patient is 5 feet 2 inches tall. Find the height of the patient in centimetres.

13. A woman weighs 165 pounds. What is her weight in kilograms?

Cumulative review exercises

Review your mastery of Chapters 1–4.

1. Convert 0.125 milligrams to micrograms.

2. 0.009 g = _____ mg

3. How many grams are contained in 5.65 kilograms?

4. 0.1 mg = _____ mcg

5. 0.06 g = _____ mg

6. 7650 mg = _____ g

7. 7.75 L = _____ mL

8. 0.6 mg = _____ mcg

9. 1250 mL = _____ L

10. Read the label in Figure C.1 and calculate the number of grams in 1 tablet of this antihistamine.

```
        Hydroxyzine hydrochloride
              10 mg tablets
```

Figure C.1 Drug label for hydroxyzine hydrochloride

11. Read the label in Figure C.2 and calculate the number of grams in 1 tablet of this antianginal drug.

```
          Nifedipine 90 mg
            100 tablets
```

Figure C.2 Drug label for nifedipine

Unit 2

Oral and parenteral medications

Chapter 5

Calculating oral medication doses

Learning outcomes

After completing this chapter, you will be able to

1. Calculate simple problems for oral medications in solid and liquid form.
2. Calculate complex problems for oral medications in solid and liquid form.
3. Interpret drug labels in order to calculate doses for oral medication.
4. Calculate doses based on body weight.
5. Calculate doses based on body surface area (BSA) using a formula or a nomogram.

The majority of medications which are prescribed, dispensed and administered are oral medications. In this chapter you will learn how to calculate doses of oral medications in solid or liquid form. You will also be introduced to problems that utilise body weight or body surface area (BSA) to calculate dosages.

Diagnostic questions

Before commencing this chapter try the following questions. Compare your answers with those in Appendix A, then work through the chapter focussing on areas where you feel unsure.

1. You wish to give your patient 1 g of paracetamol. The container indicates each tablet is 500 mg. How many tablets do you give?

2. The drug Atropine 600 mcg is to be given. How many milligrams is this?

3. Codeine 0.08 g is prescribed to a patient. How many milligrams is this?

4. A patient is to have 0.125 mg digoxin. You have a stock of digoxin 0.0625 mg. How many tablets do you give?

5. A patient is to drink one and half litres of fluid over 24 hours. How many mLs is that?

Simple problems

In the calculations you have done in previous chapters, all the equivalents have come from standard tables, for example, 100 mg = 1 g. In this chapter, the equivalent used will depend on the strength of the drug that is available; for example 1 tablet = 15 mg. In the following examples, the equivalent is found on the label of the drug container.

Medication in solid form

Example 5.1

The prescription reads *duloxetine 120 mg PO daily*. Read the drug label shown in Figure 5.1. How many capsules of this antidepressant drug will you administer to the patient?

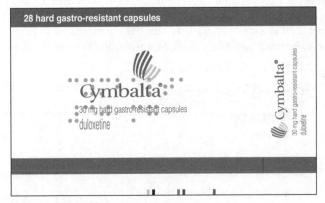

Figure 5.1 Drug label for Cymbalta

(© Eli Lilly and Company. All rights reserved. Used with permission. CYMBALTA® is a registered trademark of Eli Lilly and Company.)

Convert 120 mg to capsules:

$$120 \text{ mg} = ? \text{ cap}$$

Cancel the milligrams and calculate the equivalent amount in capsules.

$$120 \text{ mg} \times \frac{? \text{ cap}}{? \text{ mg}} = ? \text{ cap}$$

Because the label indicates that each capsule contains 30 mg, you use the unit fraction $\frac{1 \text{ cap}}{30 \text{ mg}}$:

$$\overset{4}{\cancel{120 \text{ mg}}} \times \frac{\boxed{1 \text{ cap}}}{\underset{1}{\cancel{30 \text{ mg}}}} = 4 \text{ cap}$$

So, you would give *4 capsules* by mouth once a day to the patient.

There is another way to remember the above equation for checking your calculations:

$$\frac{\text{Amount wanted}}{\text{Amount available}} \times \text{volume it is in} \left(\text{or } \frac{\text{Want}}{\text{Available}} \times \text{Volume} \right)$$

Thus, using the above example:

Amount wanted   = 120 mg

Amount available =   30 mg

Volume it is in   =   1 (capsule)

Put it in the equation: $\dfrac{120 \text{ mg}}{30 \text{ mg}} \times 1 \text{ cap} = 4 \text{ caps}$

The answer is the same: *4 capsules* by mouth once a day to the patient.

Example 5.2

A patient is prescribed *valsartan (Diovan) 120 mg PO once daily* for hypertension. Read the drug label shown in Figure 5.2 and determine how many tablets you would give to the patient.

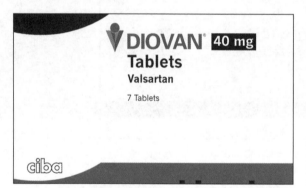

Figure 5.2 Drug label for Diovan

(Reproduced with permission of Novartis Pharmaceuticals Ltd. Sample. For educational use only.)

Convert 120 mg to tablets:

$$120 \text{ mg} = ? \text{ tab}$$

Cancel the milligrams and obtain the equivalent amount in tablets:

$$120 \text{ mg} \times \frac{? \text{ tab}}{? \text{ mg}} = ? \text{ tab}$$

Because 1 tab = 40 mg, the unit fraction is $\dfrac{1 \text{ tab}}{40 \text{ mg}}$:

$$\overset{3}{\cancel{120 \text{ mg}}} \times \frac{\boxed{1 \text{ tab}}}{\underset{1}{\cancel{40 \text{ mg}}}} = 3 \text{ tab}$$

So, you would give *3 tablets* by mouth daily to the patient.

Check this answer yourself using the other formula (Want/Available × Volume).

Example 5.3

Read the label in Figure 5.3. The prescription is for *amlodipine (Istin) 10 mg PO daily*. How many capsules of this antihypertensive drug should be administered per day?

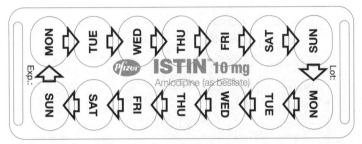

Figure 5.3 Drug label for Istin (amlodipine)
(Reprinted with permission, courtesy of Pfizer Limited)

Since the prescription requires 10 mg of amlodipine, convert the 10 mg to tablets:

$$5 \text{ mg} = ? \text{ tab}$$

Cancel the milligrams and obtain the equivalent amount in capsules:

$$10 \text{ mg} \times \frac{? \text{ tab}}{? \text{ mg}} = ? \text{ tab}$$

The label indicates that 1 tablet contains 10 mg of amlodipine. Therefore, the fraction is $\dfrac{1 \text{ tab}}{10 \text{ mg}}$:

$$\overset{1}{10 \text{ mg}} \times \frac{1 \text{ tab}}{\underset{1}{10 \text{ mg}}} = 1 \text{ tab}$$

So, you would give *1 tablet* by mouth daily to the patient.

Practice point

Some liquid oral medications are supplied with special calibrated droppers or oral syringes that are used *only* for these medications (e.g. digoxin and furosemide).

Medication in liquid form

Since paediatric and geriatric patients, as well as patients with neurological conditions, may be unable to swallow medication in tablet form, sometimes oral medications are ordered in liquid form. The label states how much drug is contained in a given amount of liquid.

Example 5.4

The physician prescribes *escitalopram (Cipramil) 10 mg PO once daily*. Read the label in Figure 5.4 and determine the number of millilitres you would administer to the patient.

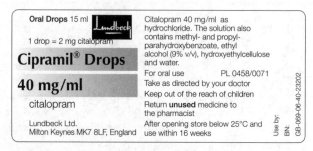

Figure 5.4 Drug label for Cipramil

(Used with permission from Lundbeck Ltd)

Convert 10 milligrams to millilitres:

$$10 \text{ mg} = ? \text{ mL}$$

Cancel the milligrams and calculate the equivalent amount in mL:

$$10 \text{ mg} \times \frac{? \text{ mL}}{? \text{ mg}} = ? \text{ mL}$$

Because the label indicates that every 1 mL of the solution contains 40 mg of escitalopram, use the unit fraction $\frac{1 \text{ mL}}{40 \text{ mg}}$:

$$10 \text{ mg} \times \frac{1 \text{ mL}}{40 \text{ mg}} = 0.25 \text{ mL}$$

So, you would give *10 mL* by mouth once a day to the patient.

Check this using the other formula (Want/Available × Volume):

Amount wanted = 10 mg

Amount available = 40 mg

Volume it is in = 1 mL

Thus it looks like this:

$$10 \text{ mg}/40 \text{ mg} \times 1 \text{ mL} = \underline{0.25 \text{ mL}}$$

Medications measured in millimoles

Some drugs such as electrolytes like potassium or sodium are measured in millimoles, which are abbreviated as mmol. Pharmaceutical companies may label electrolytes in milligrams and occasionally as milliequivalents but the latter unit is rarely used in the UK. The principles for calculating doses remain the same regardless of the unit of measurement.

Example 5.5

The prescriber orders *potassium chloride (Sando-K) 36 mmol PO daily. The box containing the potassium chloride effervescent tablets indicates that each table contains 12 mmol of potassium and 8 mmol of chloride. It is the potassium which we are most interested in and will focus on.* Determine how many tablets of this electrolyte supplement you should administer.

In this problem you want to change 36 mmol to tablets:

$$36 \text{ mmol} \longrightarrow ? \text{ tab}$$

You can do this on one line as follows:

$$36 \text{ mmol} \times \frac{? \text{ tab}}{? \text{ mmol}} = ? \text{ tab}$$

Because the label indicates that each tablet contains 12 mmol, the unit fraction is $\frac{1 \text{ tab}}{12 \text{ mmol}}$:

$$\overset{3}{\cancel{36 \text{ mmol}}} \times \frac{\boxed{1 \text{ tab}}}{\cancel{12 \text{ mmol}}} = 3 \text{ tab}$$

So, you would administer *3 tablets* of potassium chloride (Sando-K) by mouth once daily.

Check this using the other method:

Amount wanted = 36 mmol

Amount available = 12 mmol

Volume it is in = 1 tab

Thus it looks like this:

$$\frac{36 \text{ mmol}}{12 \text{ mmol}} \times 1 \text{ tab} = \underline{3 \text{ tab}}$$

Complex problems

Sometimes dosage calculations will require that multiplication by unit fractions be repeated one or more times. Recall that we examined complex problems in Chapter 3.

For example, if each tablet of a drug contains 2.5 mg, how many tablets would contain 0.0025 g? It helps to organise the information you will need for the calculation as follows:

Given quantity:	0.0025 g
Strength:	1 tab = 2.5 mg
Quantity you want to find:	? tab

You do not know the direct equivalence between grams and tablets.

This is a **complex** problem because you need to convert 0.0025 g to milligrams and then convert milligrams to tablets so there are several steps:

$$0.0025 \text{ g} \longrightarrow \text{? mg} \longrightarrow \text{? tab}$$

So, the problem is 0.0025 g = ? tab.

First, you want to cancel *grams (g)*. To do this you must use an equivalence containing *grams* to make a unit fraction with *grams* in the denominator. From the equivalence 1 g = 1000 mg, the unit fraction is $\dfrac{1000 \text{ mg}}{1 \text{ g}}$:

$$0.0025 \text{ g} \times \frac{1000 \text{ mg}}{1 \text{ g}} = \text{? tab}$$

After the *grams* are cancelled, only *milligrams* remain on the left side. Now you need to change the *milligrams* to *tablets*. From the strength 2.5 mg = 1 tab, the unit fraction is $\dfrac{1 \text{ tab}}{2.5 \text{ mg}}$:

$$0.0025 \text{ g} \times \frac{1000 \text{ mg}}{1 \text{ g}} \times \frac{1 \text{ tab}}{2.5 \text{ mg}} = \text{? tab}$$

After cancelling the milligrams, only tablets remain on the left side. Now complete your calculation by multiplying the numbers:

$$0.0025 \text{ g} \times \frac{1000 \text{ mg}}{1 \text{ g}} \times \frac{1 \text{ tab}}{2.5 \text{ mg}} = \frac{2.5 \text{ tab}}{2.5} = 1 \text{ tab}$$

So, 1 tablet contains 0.0025 g. You could also have moved the decimal point to the right to convert grams to milligrams as practised in Chapter 4 to assist with one step of this problem.

Stop and think

Be extra cautious with values less than 1 and the use of the decimal point. If in doubt always get someone else to check your calculations. It would be a responsible person who spots an error such as this on a prescription chart and points it out to the prescriber – patient safety is paramount. If you were to give a very young patient 10 mg of morphine instead of 1.0 mg that could be very dangerous – decimal points should only be used if the amount is less than 1.

Example 5.6

The prescription is *fluconazole 0.4 g PO daily*. Read the label shown in Figure 5.5 and calculate the number of tablets of this antifungal drug that should be given to the patient.

Fluconazole
100 mg tablets

Figure 5.5 Drug label for fluconazole

Given quantity: 0.4 g

Strength: 1 tab = 100 mg

Quantity you want to find: ? tab

In this problem you want to convert 0.4 g to milligrams and then convert milligrams to tablets:

$$0.4 \text{ g} \longrightarrow ? \text{ mg} \longrightarrow ? \text{ tab}$$

You can do this on one line as follows:

$$0.4 \text{ g} \times \frac{? \text{ mg}}{? \text{ g}} \times \frac{? \text{ tab}}{? \text{ mg}} = ? \text{ tab}$$

Because 1000 mg = 1 g, the first unit fraction is $\dfrac{1000 \text{ mg}}{1 \text{ g}}$.

Because 100 mg = 1 tab, the second unit fraction is $\dfrac{1 \text{ tab}}{100 \text{ mg}}$.

$$0.4 \ \cancel{g} \times \frac{\overset{10}{\cancel{1000} \text{ mg}}}{1 \ \cancel{g}} \times \frac{1 \ \boxed{\text{tab}}}{\underset{1}{\cancel{100} \text{ mg}}} = 4 \text{ tab}$$

So, you should give *4 tablets* by mouth once a day to the patient.

Note

Although Example 5.6 asks for the calculation using grams or milligrams these are used to illustrate and practise complex problems. For safety purposes, drug manufacturers often place both microgram and milligram concentrations on drug labels and prescribers should not use numbers less than 1.

Example 5.7

The prescriber orders *Norvir (ritonavir) 0.6 g PO every 12 hours*. Read the label in Figure 5.6 and determine the number of mL of this protease inhibitor your patient would receive.

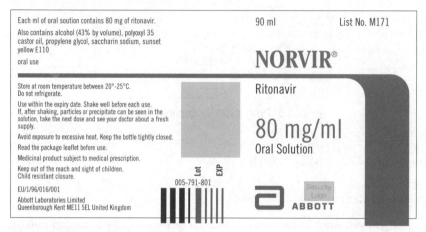

Each ml of oral soution contains 80 mg of ritonavir.

Also contains alcohol (43% by volume), polyoxyl 35 castor oil, propylene glycol, saccharin sodium, sunset yellow E110

oral use

90 ml   List No. M171

NORVIR®

Store at room temperature between 20°-25°C.
Do not refrigerate.

Use within the expiry date. Shake well before each use.
If, after shaking, particles or precipitate can be seen in the solution, take the next dose and see your doctor about a fresh supply.

Avoid exposure to excessive heat. Keep the bottle tightly closed.

Read the package leaflet before use.

Medicinal product subject to medical prescription.

Keep out of the reach and sight of children.
Child resistant closure.

EU/1/96/016/001

Abbott Laboratories Limited
Queenborough Kent ME11 5EL United Kingdom

005-791-801

Ritonavir

80 mg/ml

Oral Solution

ABBOTT

Figure 5.6 Drug label for Norvir

(Reproduced with permission of Abbott Laboratories)

Given quantity:	0.6 g
Strength:	80 mg/mL
The quantity you want to find:	? mL

In this problem you want to convert 0.6 g to milligrams and then convert milligrams to millilitres:

$$0.6 \text{ g} \longrightarrow \text{? mg} \longrightarrow \text{? mL}$$

You can do this on one line as follows:

$$0.6 \text{ g} \times \frac{\text{? mg}}{\text{? g}} \times \frac{\text{? mL}}{\text{? mg}} = \text{? mL}$$

Because 1000 mg = 1 g, the first unit fraction is $\dfrac{1000 \text{ mg}}{1 \text{ g}}$.

Because 1 mL = 80 mg, the second unit fraction is $\dfrac{1 \text{ mL}}{80 \text{ mg}}$.

$$0.6 \text{ g} \times \frac{1000 \text{ mg}}{1 \text{ g}} \times \frac{1 \text{ mL}}{80 \text{ mg}} = \frac{60}{8} \text{ mL}$$

$$= 7.5 \text{ mL}$$

So, you would give *7.5 mL* by mouth to the patient every 12 hours.

Practice point

If a prescription states 'in three divided doses,' this instructs the nurse or practitioner to separate the total daily dose into 3 equal parts over a 24–hour period. To ensure even distribution of the medication in the patient's blood stream (for optimal effect), the frequency of the doses should also be regular and consistent, so the drug is administered every 8 hours. If this were in 4 divided doses then this would be 6 hourly. This is another calculation (24 hours divided by the number of doses = time interval for doses).

Calculating dosage by body weight

Sometimes the amount of a drug is prescribed based on the patient's body weight – this is necessary with certain drugs to ensure they are effective. A patient who weighs more will receive a larger dose of the drug, and a patient who weighs less will receive a smaller dose of the drug.

Stop and think

The expression 15 mg/kg means that the patient is to receive 15 milligrams of the drug for each kilogram of body weight. Therefore, you will use the equivalent 15 mg (of drug) = 1 kg (of body weight).

Example 5.8

The prescriber prescribes 15 mg per kilogram body weight of a drug for a patient who weighs 80 kilograms. How many milligrams of this drug should the patient receive?

Body weight: 80 kg
Prescription: 15 mg/kg
Find: ? mg

Convert body weight to dosage:

$$80 \text{ kg (of body weight)} \longrightarrow \text{? mg (of drug)}$$

$$80 \text{ kg (of body weight)} \times \frac{\text{? mg (of drug)}}{\text{? kg (of body weight)}} = \text{? mg (of drug)}$$

Since the prescription is 15 mg/kg, you use the unit fraction $\dfrac{15 \text{ mg}}{1 \text{ kg}}$:

$$80 \text{ k\!g} \times \frac{15 \text{ mg}}{1 \text{ k\!g}} = 1200 \text{ mg}$$

So, the patient should receive *1200 mg* of the drug.

Example 5.9

The prescriber writes *clonazepam 0.05 mg/kg PO daily* in three divided doses for a patient who weighs 60 kilograms. If each tablet contains 1 mg, how many tablets of this anti-convulsant drug should the patient receive per day? How many tablets would the patient receive per dose?

Body weight: 60 kg
Prescription: 0.05 mg/kg
Strength: 1 tab = 1 mg
Find: ? tab

When drugs are prescribed based on body weight, you generally start the problem with the weight of the patient. You first change the single unit of measurement, kilograms (kg of body weight), to another single unit of measurement, milligrams (mg of drug), and then convert the milligrams to tablets:

$$60 \text{ kg (of body weight)} \longrightarrow ? \text{ mg (of drug)} \longrightarrow ? \text{ tab}$$

$$60 \text{ kg (of body weight)} \times \frac{? \text{ mg (of drug)}}{? \text{ kg (of body weight)}} \times \frac{? \text{ tab}}{? \text{ mg (of drug)}} = ? \text{ tab}$$

Because the prescription is for 0.05 mg per kg, the first unit fraction is $\dfrac{0.05 \text{ mg}}{1 \text{ kg}}$.

Since each tablet contains 1 mg, the second unit fraction is $\dfrac{1 \text{ tab}}{1 \text{ mg}}$.

$$60 \text{ k\!g} \times \frac{0.05 \text{ m\!g}}{1 \text{ k\!g}} \times \frac{1 \text{ tab}}{1 \text{ m\!g}} = 3 \text{ tab}$$

So, the patient should receive *3 tablets* of clonazepam by mouth *per day* in 3 divided doses; as the 24 hour day is divided in 3 this gives 8 hours so therefore the patient should receive *1 tablet* every 8 hours.

Example 5.10

The patient is prescribed *clarithromycin 7.5 mg per kilogram body weight PO b.i.d.* If the drug strength is 250 milligrams per 5 mL, how many mL of this antibiotic drug should be administered to a patient who weighs 70 kilograms?

Body weight: 70 kg

Prescription: 7.5 mg/kg

Strength: 250 mg/5 mL

Find: ? ml

Convert body weight to dosage:

$$70 \text{ kg} \longrightarrow \text{? mg} \longrightarrow \text{? mL}$$

$$70 \text{ kg} \times \frac{\text{? mg}}{\text{? kg}} \times \frac{\text{? mL}}{\text{? mg}} = \text{? mL}$$

Since the prescription specifies 7.5 mg per kg, the first fraction is $\dfrac{7.5 \text{ mL}}{\text{kg}}$.

Since the strength is 250 mg per 5 mL, the second fraction is $\dfrac{5 \text{ mL}}{250 \text{ mg}}$.

$$70 \text{ kg} \times \frac{7.5 \text{ mg}}{\text{kg}} \times \frac{5 \text{ mL}}{250 \text{ mg}} = 10.5 \text{ mL}$$

So, the patient should receive *10.5 mL* of clarithromycin by mouth 2 times per day.

Calculating dosage by body surface area

In some cases, **body surface area (BSA)** may be used rather than **weight** in determining appropriate drug dosages. This is particularly true when calculating dosages for children, the elderly and frail, those receiving cancer therapy, burn patients and patients requiring critical care. A patient's BSA can be estimated by using formulas or nomograms.

BSA formulae

BSA can be approximated by a formula using either a handheld calculator which has a function such as finding the square (n^2) or square root ($\sqrt{n}$) of a number, or an online website. BSA, which is measured in square metres (m^2), can be determined by using the following mathematical formula which is also known as the Mosteller method:

Formula for metric units:

$$BSA = \sqrt{\frac{\text{weight in kilograms} \times \text{height in centimetres}}{3600}}$$

Formula for household units:

$$BSA = \sqrt{\frac{\text{weight in pounds} \times \text{height in inches}}{3131}}$$

Example 5.11

Find the BSA of an adult who is 183 cm tall and weighs 92 kg.

Because this example has metric units (kilograms and centimetres), we use the following formula:

$$\text{BSA} = \sqrt{\frac{\text{weight in kilograms} \times \text{height in centimeters}}{3600}}$$

$$= \sqrt{\frac{92 \times 183}{3600}}$$

At this point we need a calculator with a square root key:

$$= \sqrt{4.6767}$$

$$= 2.16256$$

So, the BSA of this adult is *2.16 m²*.

Nomograms

BSA can also be approximated by using a chart called a nomogram (Figure 5.7). The nomogram includes height, weight and BSA. If a straight line is drawn on the nomogram from the patient's height (left column) to the patient's weight (right column), the line will cross the centre column at the approximate BSA of the patient. Before handheld calculators were used, the nomogram was the best tool available for determining BSA. Since electronic technology has been incorporated into most healthcare settings to ensure more accurate measurements, nomograms are becoming obsolete.

In Example 5.11 we used the formula to calculate the BSA of a person 183 cm tall, weighing 92 kg to be 2.16 m². Now let's use the adult nomogram to do the same problem. In Figure 5.8, you can see that the line from 183 cm to 92 kg crosses the BSA column at about 2.20 m².

Notice that the adult nomogram can be used to determine the BSA of patients with imperial measurements, and the resulting BSA is still in metres squared (m²) (Figure 5.9). For example, if we have a patient who is 4 ft 10 in tall and weighs 140 lbs their BSA can be determined by drawing a straight line from the height on the left (under inches) to the weight on the right (under lbs) crossing the centre BSA line giving an approximate BSA of 1.59 m².

Practice point

Whether formulae or nomograms are used to obtain BSA, the results are only approximations. This explains why we obtained both 2.16 m² (using the formula) and 2.20 m² (using the nomogram) as the BSA for the same patient in Example 5.11. Whichever method you use you must be consistent, i.e. use the calculation method all the time or the nomogram.

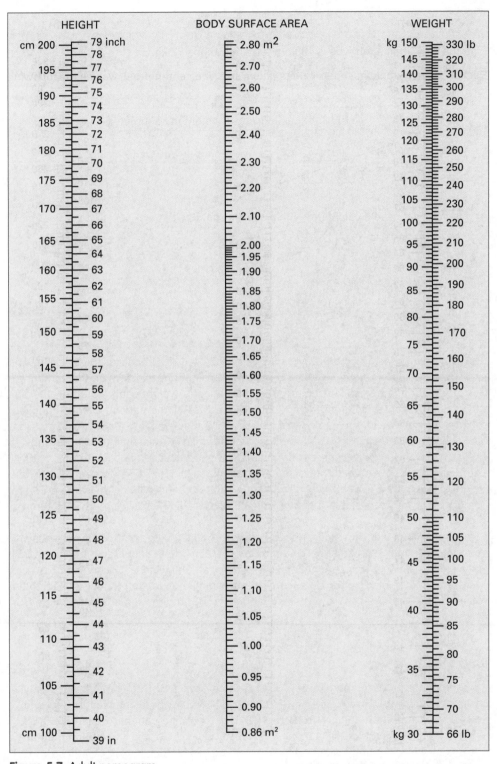

Figure 5.7 Adult nomogram

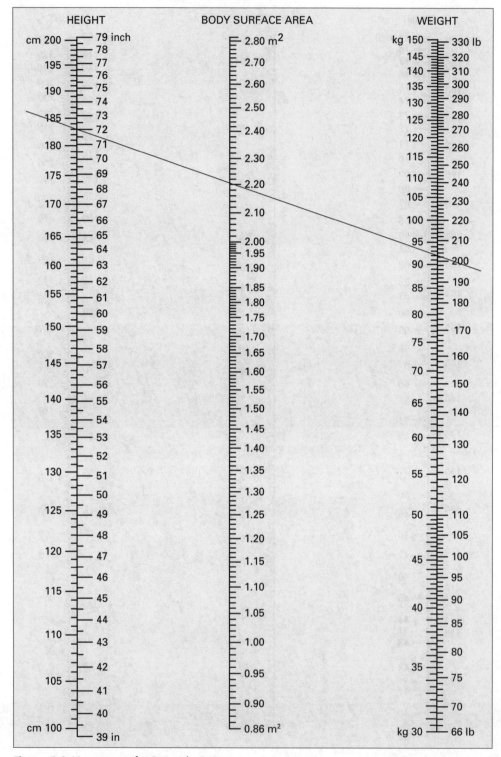

Figure 5.8 Nomogram for Example 5.11

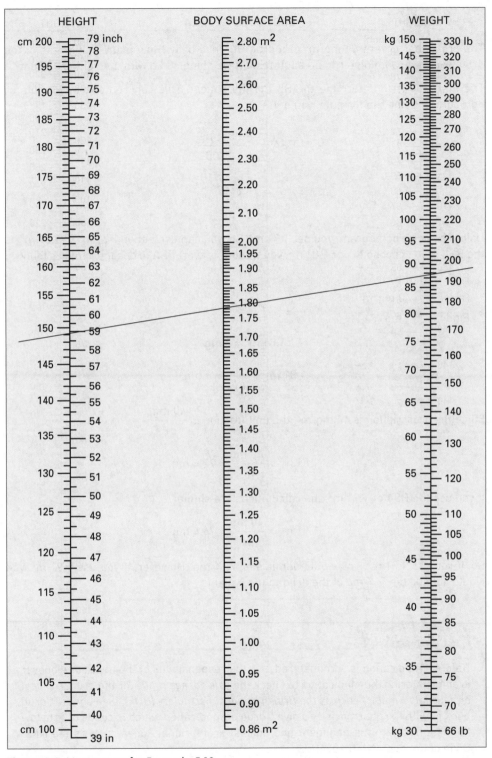

Figure 5.9 Nomogram for Example 5.12

Example 5.12

The prescriber orders 40 mg/m² of a drug PO once daily. How many milligrams of the drug would you administer to an adult patient weighing 88 kg with a height of 150 cm?

The first step is to determine the BSA of the patient. This can be done by formula or nomogram. Using the formula, you get:

$$BSA = \sqrt{\frac{88 \times 150}{3600}}$$

$$= \sqrt{3.6667}$$

$$= 1.91 \text{ m}^2$$

Using the adult nomogram, you get 1.81 m². So, you can use either 1.91 m² or 1.81 m² as the BSA. If you choose to use 1.81 m², you want to convert BSA to dosage in mg as follows:

    BSA: 1.81 m²

    Order: 40 mg/m²

    Find: ? mg

$$1.81 \text{ m}^2 = ? \text{ mg}$$

$$1.81 \text{ m}^2 \times \frac{? \text{ mg}}{\text{m}^2} = ? \text{ mg}$$

Since the prescription is 40 mg/m², the unit fraction is $\dfrac{40 \text{ mg}}{\text{m}^2}$:

$$1.81 \text{ m}^2 \times \frac{40 \text{ mg}}{\text{m}^2} = 72.4 \text{ mg}$$

If you use the BSA of 1.91 m², the calculations are similar:

$$1.91 \text{ m}^2 \times \frac{40 \text{ mg}}{\text{m}^2} = 76.4 \text{ mg}$$

So, if you use 1.81 m², you would administer 72.4 mg. However, if you use 1.91 m², you would administer *76.4 mg* of the drug to the patient.

Practice point

Before a medication is administered, it is the responsibility of the nurse or whoever is administering the medication to check the *safe dosage range* for the drug in *a local or national formulary such as the British National Formulary (BNF)*, a designated drug book or with the pharmacist. To give a drug or medication which exceeds or is below the safe dose limit is negligent and against professional codes such as the NMC Code of Conduct (NMC 2004).

Example 5.13

The prescriber orders 30 mg/m² of a drug PO stat for a patient who has a BSA of 1.65 m². The 'safe dose range' for this drug is 20–40 mg per day. Calculate the prescribed dose in milligrams and determine if it is within the safe range.

BSA: 1.65 m²

Prescription: 30 mg/m²

Find: ? mg

You want to convert the BSA of 1.65 m² to the number of milligrams ordered:

$$1.65 \text{ m}^2 = ? \text{ mg}$$

$$1.65 \text{ m}^2 \times \frac{? \text{ mg}}{\text{m}^2} = ? \text{ mg}$$

Because the prescription is 30 mg per m², the unit fraction is $\dfrac{30 \text{ mg}}{\text{m}^2}$:

$$1.65 \ \cancel{\text{m}^2} \times \frac{30 \text{ mg}}{\cancel{\text{m}^2}} = \underline{49.5 \text{ mg}}$$

The safe dose range is 20–40 mg per day. So, the dose prescribed, 49.5 mg, is higher than the upper limit (40 mg) of the daily 'safe dose range'. Therefore, the prescribed dose is *not safe*, and you would not administer this drug. You would inform the prescriber immediately and document carefully the reason for not giving the drug.

Summary

In this chapter, you learned the calculations necessary to determine dosages of oral medications in liquid and solid form.

Calculating doses for oral medications in solid and liquid form

+ The label states the strength of the drug (e.g. 10 mg/tab, 15 mg/mL).

+ Sometimes oral medications are ordered in liquid form for special populations such as paediatrics, the elderly and patients with neurological conditions.

+ Special calibrated droppers or oral syringes that are supplied with some liquid oral medications may be used to administer *only those medications*.

+ Some drugs, such as electrolytes, are measured in millimoles.

Calculating doses by body weight

+ Dosages based on body weight are generally measured in milligrams per kilo-gram(mg/kg).

+ Start calculations with the weight of the patient.

+ Medications may be prescribed by body weight in special populations such as critical care, paediatrics and elderly care.

+ It is crucial to ensure that every medication administered is within the recommended safe dosage range.

Calculating doses by body surface area

+ Body surface area (BSA) is measured in square metres (m^2).

+ Start calculations with the BSA of the patient.

+ BSA is determined by using either a formula or a nomogram.

+ BSA may be utilised to determine dosages for special patient populations such as those receiving cancer therapy, burn therapy and for patients requiring critical care.

Reference

Nursing and Midwifery Council (NMC) (2004) *The NMC code of professional conduct: standards for conduct, performance and ethics*. London: Nursing and Midwifery Council.

Case study 5.1

Mr M is a 68-year-old male patient with a past medical history of diabetes mellitus Type II and severe ischaemic cardiomyopathy. He reported that for the last 6 weeks he had been experiencing shortness of breath and fatigue at very moderate activity. He has complained of difficulty sleeping at night and has a weight gain of 5 kg, even though he described his appetite as poor. On assessment he states he does not smoke and has not had alcohol for many years as it makes him too sleepy. Whilst observing the patient the nurse notices some facial oedema especially around the eyes and bilateral pitting oedema in both lower limbs. His present weight is 70 kg and his observations are BP 160/100 mmHg, T 37 °C, slight tachycardia at P 104/min and R 28/min. Mr M was admitted for investigation and also intravenous fluid support and diuresis.

The plans for his investigations and care were as follows:

Investigations: Full blood count

+ Complete blood test for urea and electrolytes, liver function tests and blood glucose

+ Coronary angiogram; ECG; stress perfusion scan; chest X-ray

Care plan:

+ Monitor activities and support with all activities of daily living where the patient is having difficulty

+ Monitor dietary sodium intake and referral to a dietition: Low-salt diet (2 g/day)

+ Monitor fluid balance: daily weight at 07.30, strict recording of fluid intake and output

The doctor prescribes a series of drugs which include:

+ furosemide (Lasix) 80 mg PO stat
+ furosemide (Lasix) 60 mg PO 12 hourly to begin 12 hours after the stat dose
+ digoxin 0.25 mg PO once daily
+ potassium chloride (Sando-K) 24 mmol PO daily
+ chlorpropamide (Diabinese) 125 mg PO each morning with breakfast
+ docusate sodium (Docusol) 100 mg PO t.i.d.
+ lorazepam (Ativan) 3 mg PO nocte
+ fluid restriction 1500 mL/24 h

1. The patient drank 650 mL of H_2O, 150 mL of cranberry juice and 200 mL of ginger ale during the 7 a.m. to 7 p.m. shift. How many mL of fluid may the patient be given over the next 12 hours?

2. At 8 p.m., Mr M's wife fed him 375 mL of an organic brand of chicken broth, which contains 390 mg salt in each 250 mL serving.

   (a) How many grams of salt did he consume?

   (b) How much more salt should Mr M consume for the remainder of the day?

3. The diuretic drug furosemide (Lasix) is available in 20 mg tablets.

   (a) How many tablets will you administer for the stat dose?

   (b) How many tablets will the patient have received within the first 20 hours?

4. How many millimoles of the electrolyte supplement potassium chloride will the patient have received after 5 days of therapy?

5. Docusate sodium, a stool-softening drug, is supplied as an oral liquid, 20 mg/5 mL.

   (a) How many times a day does the patient receive this medication?

   (b) How many mL would the patient receive in two days?

6. The available strength of lorazepam (Ativan) is 1 mg/tab. How many tablets of this sedative contain the prescribed dose?

7. The cardiac drug Digoxin is supplied in the following strengths: 50 mcg, 100 mcg and 200 mcg tablets. Which combination of tablets would yield the least number of tablets that would deliver the prescribed dose?

8. Mr M remains hospitalised for one week. How many milligrams of chlorpropamide would he have received by the end of the first 7 days?

Practice reading labels

Calculate the following doses using the labels shown. You will find the answers in Appendix A in the back of the book.

Metoprolol tartrate
50 mg tablets
Expiry December 2010
Protect from moisture
Dispense in tight, light-resistant
container

Bupropion hydrochloride
Tablets
100 mg

1. Metoprolol
0.05 g = _____ tab

2. Bupropion hydrochloride
200 mg = _____ tab

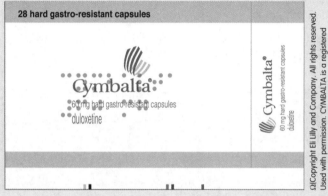

3. Cymbalta (duloxetine HCl) 0.12 g = _____ cap

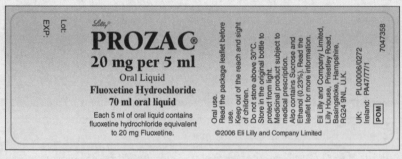

4. Prozac (fluoxetine) 40 mg = _____ mL

Erythromycin
250 mg
Tablets

Imatinib mesilate
400 mg tablets

5. Erythromycin 0.25 g = _____ tab

6. Imatinib mesylate 800 mg = _____ tab

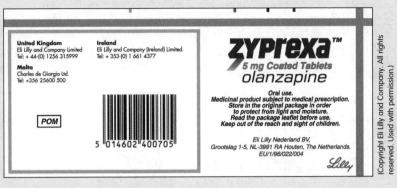

7. Zyprexa (olanzapine) 10 mg = _____ tab

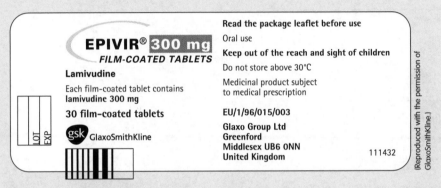

8. Epivir (lamivudine) 0.6 g = _____ tab

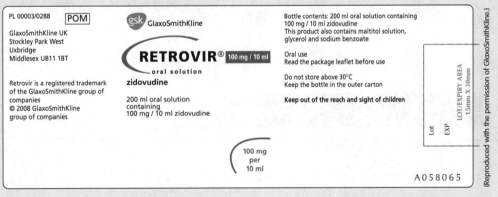

9. Retrovir (zidovudine) 100 mg = _____ mL

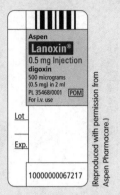

(Reproduced with permission from Aspen Pharmacare.)

Aspen
Lanoxin®
0.5 mg Injection
digoxin
500 micrograms
(0.5 mg) in 2 ml
PL 35468/0001 POM
For i.v. use

Lot

Exp.

10000000067217

10. Lanoxin (digoxin)
125 mcg = _____ mL

Metoprolol succinate
200 mg tablets

11. Metoprolol succinate
0.4 g = _____ tab

Felodipine tablets
2.5 mg

12. Felodipine SR 5 mg = _____ tab

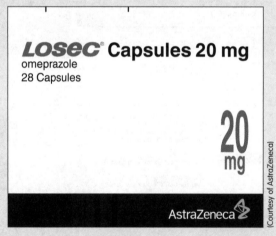

LOSEC® Capsules 20 mg
omeprazole
28 Capsules

20
mg

AstraZeneca

(Courtesy of AstraZeneca)

13. Losec (omeprazole) 80 mg = _____ cap

Metoprolol tartrate
injection
5 mg in 5 mL

14. Lopresor (metoprolol) 0.05 mg = _____ mL

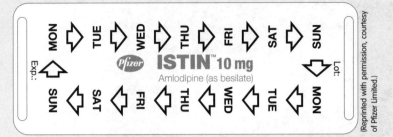

(Reprinted with permission, courtesy of Pfizer Limited.)

15. Istin (amlodipine) 10 mg = _____ cap

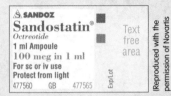

(Reproduced with the permission of Novartis Pharmaceuticals.)

16. Sandostatin (octreotide) 0.1 mg = _____ mL

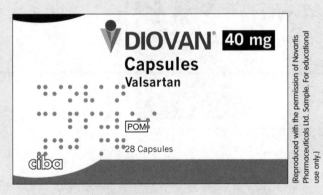

(Reproduced with the permission of Novartis Pharmaceuticals Ltd. Sample. For educational use only.)

17. Diovan (valsartan) 0.08 g = _____ tab

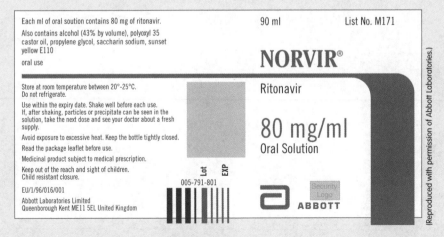

(Reproduced with permission of Abbott Laboratories.)

18. Norvir (ritonavir) 130 mg = _____ mL

115

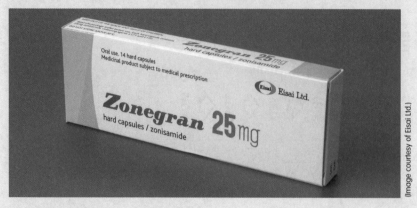

(Image courtesy of Eisai Ltd.)

19. Zonegran (zonisamide) 75 mg = _____ cap

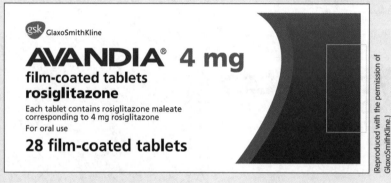

(Reproduced with the permission of GlaxoSmithKline.)

20. Avandia (rosiglitazone) 8 mg = _____ tab

Practice sets

The answers to *Try these for practice* and *Exercises* appear in Appendix A at the end of the book.

Try these for practice

Test your comprehension after reading the chapter.

1. The prescription is *quinapril HCl (Accupro) 40 mg PO b.i.d.*

   (a) Read the label in Figure 5.10 to determine how many tablets of this antihypertensive drug you will administer.

   (b) Express the daily dose in grams.

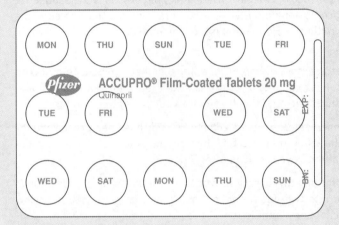

Figure 5.10 Drug label for Accupro
(Reprinted with permission, courtesy of Pfizer Limited)

2. The prescriber requests *Methotrexate 25 mg/m² PO twice per week* to treat leukemia. How many milligrams would you administer in one week if the patient is 150 cm tall and weighs 70 kg?

3. A prescription reads *Pregabalin 50 mg PO t.i.d.* The bottle contains 25 mg capsules. How many capsules of this anticonvulsive medication would you administer in 24 hours?

4. The prescriber prescribes *Thioridazine HCl 80 mg PO t.i.d.* for a patient with schizophrenia. If you have 10, 15 and 50 mg non-scored tablets to chose from, which combination of tablets would contain the exact dosage with the smallest number of tablets?

```
Metoprolol succinate
200 mg tablets
Expiry December 2010
Protect from moisture
Dispense in tight, light-resistant
container
```

Figure 5.11 Drug label for metoprolol

(Exercises)

Reinforce your understanding in class or at home.

1. *Paroxetine HCl 40 mg PO daily* has been ordered for your patient. Each tablet contains 0.02 g. How many tablets of this antidepressant will you prepare?

2. The physician prescribes *500 mcg of entecavir (Baraclude) per day* via NG (nasogastric tube) for a patient with chronic hepatitis B virus infection. The oral solution contains 0.05 mg of entecavir per millilitre. How many mL of this antiviral medication would you deliver?

3. The prescriber prescribes *acarbose 75 mg PO t.i.d.* for a diabetic patient to be taken with meals. The medication is available in 25 mg tablets. How many tablets of this α glucosidase inhibitor (antidiabetic agent) will you give your patient in 24 hours?

4. *Metoprolol succinate extended-release tablets 200 mg PO daily* has been prescribed for a patient. After reading the label in Figure 5.11 how many tablets of this antihypertensive drug would the patient have received after 7 days?

5. Cephalexin is prescribed for an elderly patient who weighs 40 kg. The prescription is *50 mg/kg daily PO* divided into two equal doses. Each tablet contains 500 mg. How many tablets of this cephalosporin antibiotic will the patient receive per dose?

6. A patient is scheduled to receive 0.015 g of a drug by mouth every morning. The drug is available as 7.5 mg tablets. How many tablets would you administer?

7. A patient with osteoarthritis is prescribed *Voltarol (diclofenac sodium) 150 mg PO per day* in 3 divided doses. There are 25 mg tablets available. How many tablets will you give in a single dose?

8. A patient develops a mild skin reaction to a transfusion of a unit of packed red blood cells and is given *75 mg of diphenhydramine HCl (Benadryl) PO stat*. The only drug strength available is 25 mg capsules. How many capsules will you give?

9. The doctor prescribes *warfarin sodium 6.5 mg PO every other day* from Monday to Sunday. How many milligrams of warfarin will your patient receive in that week?

10. The antibiotic, Zithromax (azithromycin), is ordered to treat a patient with a bacterial exacerbation of chronic obstructive pulmonary disease (COPD). The prescription is *Zithromax (azithromycin) 500 mg PO as a single dose on day one, followed by 250 mg once daily on days 2 to 5*: How many milligrams will the patient receive by the completion of the prescription?

Syringes

After completing this chapter, you will be able to

1. Identify various types of syringes.

2. Read and measure dosages on syringes.

3. Read the calibrations on hypodermic, insulin and prefilled syringes.

4. Measure single insulin dosages.

In this chapter, you will learn how to use various types of syringes to measure medication dosages. You will also discuss the difference between the types of insulin and how to measure single insulin dosages.

Syringes are made of plastic or glass, designed for one-time use and are packaged either separately or together with needles of appropriate sizes. After use, syringes must be discarded in special puncture-resistant containers adhering to local and legislative (Health and Safety) sharps disposal procedures.

Diagnostic questions

Before commencing this chapter try the following questions. Compare your answers with those in Appendix A.

1. List three types of injection routes.

2. A patient is to have 25 units of insulin. The stock insulin is 100 units per mL. Do you draw up the insulin in any syringe as mLs or do you use a specific syringe?

3. A patient is being prepared for surgery and due to have an injection of Atropine 600 mcg. You need to draw up 0.6 mL. What is the best syringe to use: 1 mL, 2 mL, 5 mL, 10 mL?

4. If a patient is prescribed 2 types of insulin can they be drawn up in the same syringe?

5. In what way can syringes cause drug errors?

Parts of a syringe

A syringe consists of a barrel, plunger and tip.

+ **Barrel:** a hollow cylinder that holds the medication. It has calibrations (markings) on the outer surface.
+ **Plunger:** fits in the barrel and is moved back and forth. Pulling back on the plunger draws medication or air into the syringe. Pushing in the plunger forces air or medication out of the syringe.
+ **Tip:** the end of the syringe that holds the needle. The needle slips onto the tip or can be twisted and locked in place (Luer-lock).

The inside of the barrel, plunger and tip (shown in Figure 6.1) must always be sterile.

Needles

Needles are made of stainless steel and come in various lengths and diameters. They are packaged with a protective cover that keeps them from being contaminated. The parts of a needle are the **hub**, which attaches to the syringe, the **shaft**, the long part of the needle that is embedded in the hub, and the **bevel**, the slanted portion of the tip. The **length** of the needle is the distance from the point to the hub. Needles most commonly

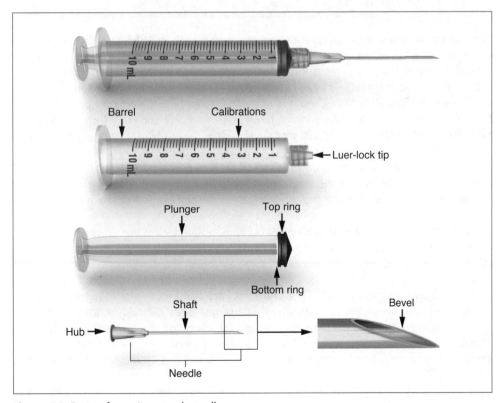

Figure 6.1 Parts of a syringe and needle

used in medication administration range from 2 to 5 cm in length. The **gauge** of the needle refers to the thickness of the inside of the needle and varies from 18 to 28 (the larger the gauge, the thinner the needle). The parts of a needle are shown in Figure 6.1.

Practice point

The patient's size, the type of tissue being injected and the viscosity (thickness) of the medication will determine the size of the needle to be used. The inside of the barrel, plunger, tip of the syringe, and the needle should never come in contact with anything unsterile. Do link this with your knowledge of injection techniques and aseptic techniques.

Stop and think

If you feel unfamiliar with syringes remember – there are only three parts to a syringe – they come in different sizes but all are essentially the same.

Types of syringes

The two major types of syringes are hypodermic and oral. In 1853, Drs Charles Pravaz and Alexander Wood were the first to develop a syringe with a needle that was fine enough to pierce the skin. This is known as a **hypodermic syringe**. (Use of oral syringes will be discussed in Chapter 11.) In recent years syringes have been the source of drug errors (Smith 2004; RCN 2006) and it is best for the nurse or healthcare practitioner to be familiar with the parts of the syringe, how to use a syringe and the difference between syringes. Increasingly, syringes will be colour coded to identify oral from parenteral use syringes. It has also been suggested that syringes are manufactured to ensure that they have unique locking systems so a medication prepared in a parenteral syringe cannot accidentally be used to give the medication through a different route (i.e. giving intravenous drugs in error through the intrathecal route) and be potentially harmful to the patient (Smith 2004).

Hypodermic syringes are calibrated (marked) in millilitres (mL) or units. Practitioners often refer to syringes by the volume they contain, for example, a 5 mL syringe. The term mL instead of cc will be used when referring to syringes; this latter term may be seen in older texts or texts from overseas.

The smaller capacity syringes (1, 2 and 3 mL) are used most often for subcutaneous or intramuscular injections of medication. The larger sizes (5 or 10 mL) are commonly used to withdraw blood or prepare medications for intravenous administration. Syringes 20 mL and larger are used to inject large volumes of sterile solutions. A representative sample of commonly used syringes is shown in Figure 6.2. A 10 mL syringe is shown in Figure 6.3. Each line on the barrel represents 0.2 mL and the longer lines represent 1 mL. A 5 mL syringe is shown in Figure 6.4. Each line on the barrel represents 0.2 mL, and the longer lines represent 1 mL.

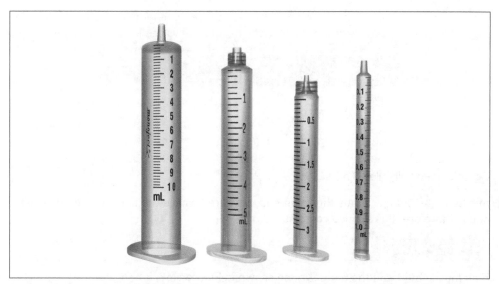

Figure 6.2 A sample of commonly used hypodermic syringes (10 mL, 5 mL, 3 mL and 1 mL)

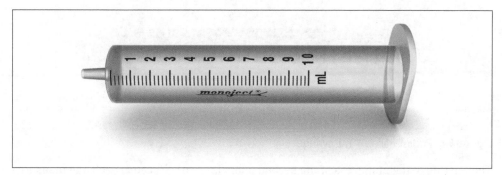

Figure 6.3 10 mL syringe

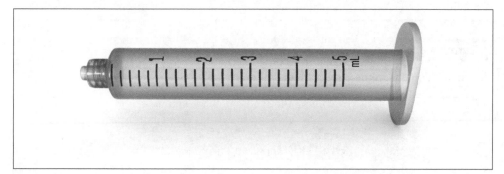

Figure 6.4 5 mL syringe

In Figure 6.5, a syringe is shown which has 10 spaces between the largest markings. This indicates that the syringe is measured in tenths of a millilitre. So, each of the lines is 0.1 mL. The longer lines indicate half and full millilitre measures. The liquid volume in a syringe is read from the *top ring*, **not** the bottom ring or the raised section in the

123

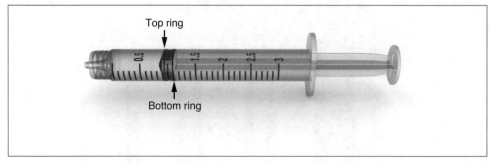

Figure 6.5 Partially filled 3 mL syringe

middle of the plunger. Thus the volume is measured where the liquid meets the rubber bung. Therefore, this syringe contains 0.9 mL.

Example 6.1

How much liquid is in the 5 mL syringe shown in Figure 6.6?

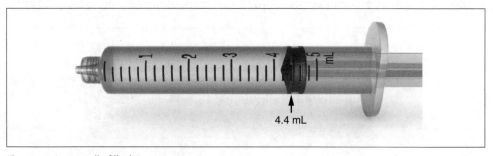

Figure 6.6 Partially filled 5 mL syringe

The top ring of the plunger is at the second line after 4 mL. Because each line measures 0.2 mL, the second line measures 0.4 mL. Therefore, the amount of liquid in the syringe is 4.4 mL.

Example 6.2

How much liquid is in the 3 mL syringe in Figure 6.7?

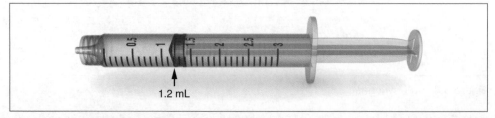

Figure 6.7 Partially filled 3 mL syringe

The top ring of the plunger is at the second line after 1 mL. Because each line measures 0.1 mL, the two lines measure 0.2 mL. Therefore, the amount in the syringe is 1.2 mL.

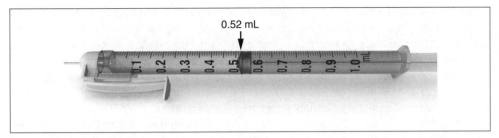

Figure 6.8 Partially filled 1 mL tuberculin syringe

The 1 mL syringe, also called a **tuberculin syringe**, shown in Figure 6.8, is calibrated in hundredths of a millilitre. Because there are 100 lines on the syringe, each line represents 0.01 mL. This syringe is used for intradermal injection of very small amounts of substances in tests for tuberculosis and allergies, as well as for intramuscular injection of small quantities of medication. The top ring of the plunger is at the second line after 0.5 mL. Therefore, the amount in the syringe is 0.52 mL.

Example 6.3

How much liquid is shown in the portion of the 1 mL tuberculin syringe shown in Figure 6.9?

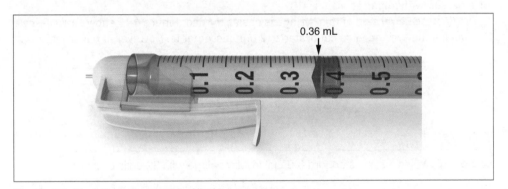

Figure 6.9 A portion of a partially filled 1 mL syringe

The top ring of the plunger is 6 lines after the 0.3 mL calibration. Because each line represents 0.01 mL, the amount of liquid in the syringe is 0.36 mL.

Note

Because the 1 mL tuberculin syringe can accurately measure amounts to hundredths of a millilitre, the volume of fluid to be measured in this syringe is rounded up or down to the nearest hundredth (i.e. 2 decimal places); for example, 0.358 mL is rounded up to 0.36 mL. The 3 mL syringe can accurately measure amounts to tenths of a millilitre. The volume of fluid to be measured in this syringe is rounded up or down to the nearest tenth of a millilitre; for example, 2.35 mL is rounded up to 2.4 mL.

Insulin syringes are used for the subcutaneous injection of insulin and are calibrated in *units* rather than *millilitres*. Insulin is a hormone used to treat patients who have Type 1 diabetes mellitus (previously known as insulin-dependent diabetes mellitus). It is supplied as a premixed liquid measured in standardised units of potency rather than by weight or volume. These standardised units are called **USP** *units*, which are often shortened to *units*. This term should always be written in full on prescription charts to avoid confusion. The most commonly prepared concentration of insulin is 100 units per millilitre, which is referred to as *units 100 insulin* and is abbreviated as U-100 on insulin labels. Although a 500 unit concentration of insulin (U-500) is also available, it is used only for the rare patient who is markedly insulin-resistant. Exubera, the first inhalable version of insulin, is available as a dry powder and is inhaled through the mouth using the handheld Exubera Inhaler. This is a significant development, but is not yet as widely used or evaluated against injectable insulin and at present is not recommended for diabetic patients (NICE 2006). This has a clear advantage for injection-phobic patients, however, injectable insulin remains the main approach. For the remainder of this chapter, we will refer to the standard 100 unit insulin only.

Insulin syringes have three different capacities: the standard 100 unit and the 50 unit capacities. The plunger of the insulin syringe is flat, and the liquid volume is measured from the top ring.

Figure 6.10 shows a *single-scale standard* 100 unit insulin syringe calibrated in 2 unit increments. Any odd number of units (e.g. 23, 35) is measured between the even calibrations. These calibrations and spaces are very small, so this is not the syringe of choice for a person with impaired vision.

The dual-scale version of this syringe is easier to read. Figure 6.11 shows a *dual-scale* 100 unit insulin syringe, also calibrated in 2 unit increments. However, it has a scale with

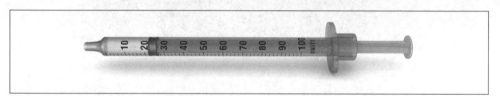

Figure 6.10 A single-scale standard 100 unit insulin syringe with 22 units of insulin

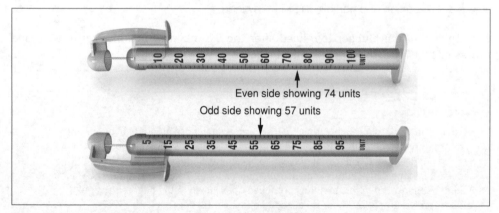

Figure 6.11 Two views of the same dual-scale standard 100 unit insulin syringe

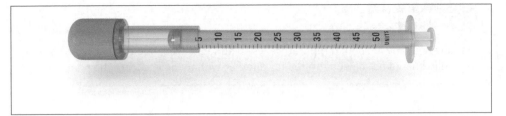

Figure 6.12 A 50 unit Lo-Dose insulin syringe

even numbers on one side and a scale with *odd* numbers on the opposite side. Both the even and odd sides are shown. Each line on the barrel represents 2 units.

A 50 unit insulin syringe, shown in Figure 6.12, is a single-scale syringe with 50 units. It is calibrated in 1 unit increments.

Stop and think

Don't panic – think carefully about the main numbers on a syringe – if the main numbers are 1 and then 2, then look in between, count the smaller markings. If there are 10 of these, the units are 1/10th or 0.1 increments. If there are 5 smaller markings, then the units are 1/5th or 0.2 increments. To familiarise yourself with these look on a standard measuring ruler – see the markings between the 1 and 2 cm marks – these are millimetres and there are 10 of them – so 1 cm is followed by 1.1, then 1.2, then 1.3 and so on until 1.9 then you reach 2 cm.

Stop and think

Insulin is always ordered in units, the medication is supplied in 100 units/mL and the syringes are calibrated for 100 units/mL. Therefore, no calculations are required to prepare insulin that is administered subcutaneously.

The insulin syringe is to be used in the measurement and administration of 100 units/mL insulin *only*. It must not be used to measure other medications that are also measured in units, such as heparin.

Practice point

Select the appropriate syringe and be very attentive to the calibrations when measuring insulin dosages. Both the single- and dual-scale standard 100 unit insulin syringes are calibrated in 2 unit increments. The 50 unit syringes are calibrated in 1 unit increments.

Practice point

Insulin should be at room temperature when administered, and one source or brand of insulin should not be substituted for another without advice from the pharmacist.

Measuring insulin doses

Measuring a single dose of insulin in an insulin syringe

Insulin is available in 100 units/mL multidose vials. The major route of administration of insulin is by subcutaneous injection. *Insulin is never given intramuscularly*. It can also be administered with an insulin pen that contains a cartridge filled with insulin or with a CSII pump (Continuous Subcutaneous Insulin Infusion). The CSII pump is used to administer a programmed dose of a rapid-acting 100 units insulin at a set rate of units per hour.

The **source** of insulin (animal or human) and **type** (rapid, short, intermediate or long-acting) are indicated on the label. Today, the most commonly used *source* is human insulin. Insulin from a human source is designated on the label as recombinant DNA (rDNA origin). The *type* of insulin relates to both the *onset and duration of action*. It is indicated by the uppercase bold letter that follows the trade name on the label, for example, **Humulin S (Regular), Humulin I (intermediate), Humulin M3 (mixed)**. These letters are important visual identifiers when selecting the insulin type (see Figure 6.13).

Healthcare providers must be familiar with the various *types of insulin*, though caution should be made as names and manufacturers of insulin, as with all drugs, will vary over time. Do ensure you familiarise yourself with any insulins to be used – some are summarised in Table 6.1.

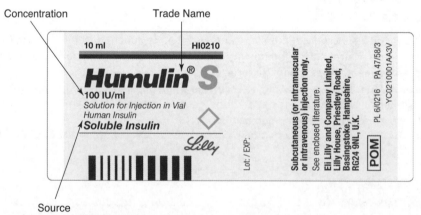

Figure 6.13 Drug label for Humulin S (Actrapid) insulin

Table 6.1 Types of insulin

Type	Name		How It Works
Rapid-acting (generic)	Humalog (Lispro)	Apidra (Glulisine)	Rapid-acting insulin covers insulin needs for meals eaten at the time of injection. Usually taken 15 minutes before meals or given just after a meal. This type of insulin is also given to cover until longer-acting insulins take effect.
Onset	15–30 minutes	10–20 minutes	
Peak	30 minutes–2½ hours	1–1½ hours	
Duration	3–5 hours	2–5 hours	
Short-acting (regular)	Humulin S	Novo-rapid	Short-acting insulin covers insulin needs for meals eaten within 30–60 minutes. Usually taken 30 to 40 minutes before meals.
Onset	30 minutes–1 hour	10–20 minutes	
Peak	2–6 hours	1–3 hours	
Duration	5–8 hours	3–5 hours	
Intermediate-acting	Insulatard or NPH	Hypurin (NB Bovine insulin)	Intermediate-acting insulin covers insulin needs for about half the day or overnight. Taken up to 1 hour before meals. This type of insulin is often combined with rapid- or short-acting insulin.
Onset	2–4 hours	1–2½ hours	
Peak	4–12 hours	6–12 hours	
Duration	14–16 hours	12–18 hours	
Long-acting and biphasic	Levenir	Lantus (glargine)	Long-acting insulin covers insulin needs for about 1 full day, not timed to meals. Some are given once or twice daily, and others once a day. Lantus once a day should be given at the same time. This type of insulin is often combined, when needed, with rapid- or short-acting insulin.
Onset	30 minutes–3 hours	1–1½ hours	
Peak	Peakless	No peak time; insulin is delivered at a steady level	
Duration	20–36 hours	20–24 hours	

Mixed insulins – these are a premixed combination of medium- and short-acting insulins

Mixed analogues – these are a premixed combination of medium-acting insulin and a short-acting analogue (insulin like product)

Premixed	Humulin M3 70/30	Novomix 30 70/30	Humalog mix 50 50/50	Humalog mix 25 75/25	Premixed insulin is a combination of specific proportions of intermediate-acting and short-acting insulin. The numbers after the name indicate the percentage of each insulin. These products are generally taken twice a day before mealtime, 15–45 minutes before meals.
Onset	30 minutes	30 minutes	30 minutes	15 minutes	
Peak	2–4 hours	2–12 hours	2–5 hours	30 minutes–2½ hours	
Duration	14–24 hours	up to 24 hours	18–24 hours	16–20 hours	

Sources: BNF (2008), Electronic Medicines Compendium http://www.emc.medicines.org

Example 6.4

What is the dose of insulin in the single-scale 1.0 mL, 100 unit insulin syringe shown in Figure 6.14?

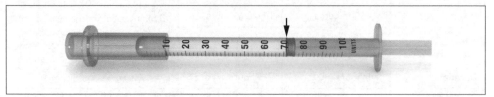

Figure 6.14 A single-scale 100 unit insulin syringe

The top ring of the plunger is one line after 70. Because each line represents 2 units, the dose is *72 units*.

Example 6.5

What is the dose of insulin in the 0.5 mL (or 50 unit) insulin syringe shown in Figure 6.15?

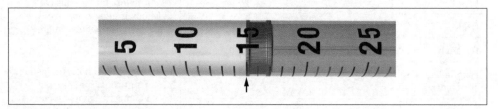

Figure 6.15 A 50 unit insulin syringe

The top ring of the plunger is at 15. Because each line represents 1 unit, the dose is *15 units*.

Example 6.6

What is the dose of insulin in the 0.5 mL (or 50 unit) insulin syringe shown in Figure 6.16?

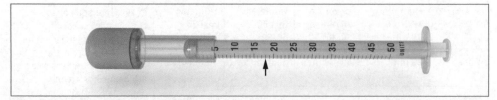

Figure 6.16 A 50 unit Lo-Dose insulin syringe

The top ring of the plunger is three lines after 15. Because each line represents one unit, the dose is *18 units*.

Example 6.7

A patient is prescribed 26 units of Humulin I insulin subcutaneously before breakfast. Read the label in Figure 6.17 to identify the source of the insulin and place an arrow at the appropriate level of measurement on the insulin syringe in Figure 6.18.

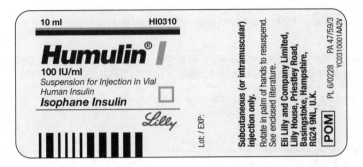

Figure 6.17 Drug label for Humulin I

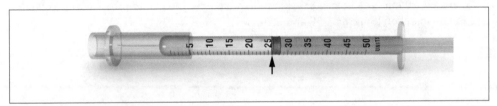

Figure 6.18 Insulin syringe for Example 6.7

The source of the insulin is human (rDNA origin), and the arrow should be placed one line after 25, as shown in Figure 6.18.

Measuring two types of insulin in one syringe

Individuals who have type 1 diabetes mellitus (formerly known as Insulin Dependent Diabetes Mellitus) often must have two types of insulin administered at the same time. In order to reduce the number of injections, it is possible to combine two insulins (usually a rapid-acting with either an intermediate- or a long-acting) in a single syringe. In general, this is not commonplace as premixed insulins are widely available. However, there are situations such as in the community where this may still be performed (RCN 2007). The important points to remember then are:

+ The *total volume* in the syringe is the *sum of the two insulin* amounts.
+ The smallest capacity syringe containing the dose should be used to measure the insulins because the enlarged scale is easier to read and therefore more accurate.
+ The *amount of air equal to the amount of insulin to be withdrawn* from each vial must be injected into each vial.
+ You must inject the air into the intermediate- or long-acting insulin before you inject the air into the Regular insulin.

131

+ The *Regular* (rapid-acting) insulin is drawn up *first*; this prevents contamination of the Regular insulin with the intermediate insulin (Diabetes UK 2008).

+ The intermediate-acting or long-acting insulins can precipitate; therefore, they must be mixed well before drawing up and administered without delay.

+ Only insulins from the same source should be mixed together; for example, Insulatard and Actrapid are both human insulin and can be mixed.

+ If you draw up too much of the intermediate insulin, you must discard the entire medication and start over.

+ Long acting insulins such as Levemir or Lantus are not suitable for mixing and guidance from the pharmacist should be sought if unsure (RCN, 2007).

The steps of preparing two types of insulin in one syringe are shown in Example 6.8.

Example 6.8

A patient is prescribed 10 units Actrapid insulin and 30 units Insulatard insulin subcutaneously, 30 minutes before breakfast. Explain how you would prepare to administer this in one injection (Figures 6.19 and 6.20).

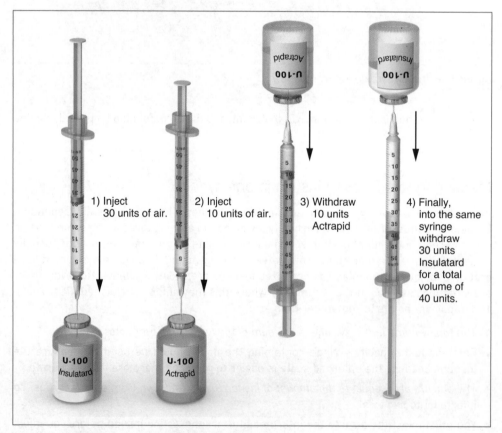

Figure 6.19 Mixing two types of insulin in one syringe

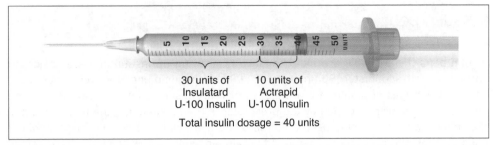

30 units of   10 units of
Insulatard   Actrapid
U-100 Insulin   U-100 Insulin

Total insulin dosage = 40 units

Figure 6.20 Combination of 30 units of Insulatard and 10 units of Actrapid

The total amount of insulin is 40 units (10 + 30). To administer this dose, use a 50 unit syringe. Inject 30 units of air into the Insulatard vial and 10 units of air into the Actrapid vial. Withdraw 10 units of the Actrapid first and then withdraw 30 units of the Insulatard.

Measuring premixed insulin

Using premixed insulin (see Table 6.1) eliminates errors that may occur when mixing two types of insulin in one syringe (Figure 6.19).

Example 6.9

Order: Give 35 units of Humulin M3 70/30 insulin subcutaneously 30 minutes before breakfast. Use the label shown in Figure 6.21 and place an arrow at the appropriate calibration on the syringe.

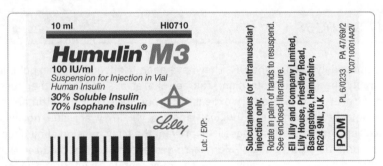

Figure 6.21 Drug label for Humulin M3 70/30

In the syringe in Figure 6.22, the top ring of the plunger is at the 35 unit line.

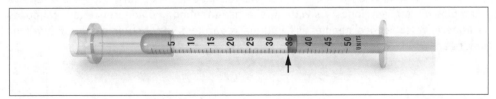

Figure 6.22 A 50 unit Lo-Dose insulin syringe measuring 35 units

Insulin pens

Insulin pens (Figure 6.23) are an alternative to drawing up insulin and are easier for patients to self-administer (Summers *et al.* 2004). Depending upon the type of pen used, specific cartridges of insulin are available which are inserted into the pen device. The dosage required or prescribed by the prescriber is then dialled into the pen device and the patient can then inject himself or herself. There are cautions, namely disposal of the used needles and cartridges. The need to maintain vigilance for signs of altered blood sugar (i.e. hypoglycaemia) and to seek advice must be emphasised to patients. There are even devices available for patients with 'needle phobia' which are not injectable but work via high-pressure air flow forcing insulin through the skin – for more information visit the Diabetes UK website.

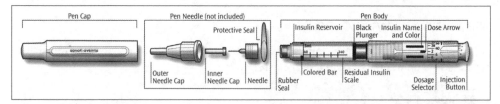

Figure 6.23 Insulin pen

(Diagram reprinted with kind permission from sanofi-aventis)

Safety syringes

These are not widely used in the UK. They have been trialled in a variety of clinical situations, namely the dental profession (Zakrzewska *et al.* 2001) and their use is being evaluated. At present they are very expensive to purchase, but the ultimate cost to the profession and health service is unclear and, as yet, they are still not widely seen. The main advantage of safety syringes is to prevent the transmission of bloodborne infections from contaminated needles. Many syringes are now manufactured with various types of safety devices. For example, a syringe may contain an integral protective sheath that can be used to protect the needle's sterility. This sheath is then pulled forward and locked into place to provide a permanent needle shield for disposal following injection. Others may have a needle that automatically retracts into the barrel after injection.

Each of these devices reduces the chance of needle stick injury. Figure 6.24 shows examples of safety syringes. As with all sharps, attention and adherence to local policy is imperative to reduce needlestick injuries regardless of whether safety syringes or others are used.

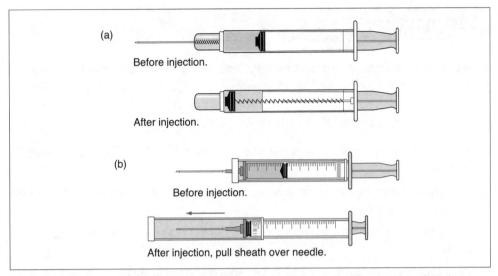

(a)

Before injection.

After injection.

(b)

Before injection.

After injection, pull sheath over needle.

Figure 6.24 Safety syringes with (a) a passive safety device and (b) an active safety device

Stop and think

When preparing an injection do think about:

+ the appropriate syringe for the medication (size or drug specific such as insulin)
+ markings or units of measurements for the medication and on the syringe
+ the appropriate needles to use (for intramuscular or subcutaneous injections)
+ which parts of the syringe and needle are sterile and should be kept that way

Link this to your knowledge of how to give injections.

Practice point

Do be careful and think of what can go wrong: a young nurse is preparing an insulin injection for a patient, she cannot find a small insulin syringe like the one she used yesterday with her mentor and so decides she can use a 5 mL syringe. She draws up 30 units of Actrapid insulin (100 units/mL) and checks this with her mentor who sees she has drawn up 3 mL insulin. She is stopped immediately as she would be giving the patient 300 units of insulin not 30; this could have had serious consequences for a patient (and the nurse). The moral – if the equipment is not obviously there ask for help!

Summary

In this chapter, the various types of syringes and needles were discussed. You learned how to measure the amount of liquid in various syringes. The types of insulin, how to measure a single dose, and how to mix two insulins in one syringe were explained. Prefilled, single-dose and safety syringes were also presented.

+ Millilitres (mL) rather than cubic centimetres (cc) are the preferred unit of measure for volume.

+ All syringe calibrations must be read at the top ring of the plunger, i.e. where the plunger meets the liquid.

+ Large-capacity hypodermic syringes (5, 10, 20, 35 mL) are calibrated in increments from 0.2 mL to 1 mL.

+ Small-capacity hypodermic syringes (2, 3 mL) are calibrated in tenths of a millilitre (0.1 mL).

+ The calibrations on hypodermic syringes differ; therefore, be very careful when measuring medications in syringes.

+ Insulin syringes are designed for measuring and administering U-100 insulin. They are calibrated for 100 units per mL.

+ Standard insulin syringes have a capacity of 100 units.

+ Smaller insulin syringes are used for measuring small amounts of insulin. They have a capacity of 50 units (0.5 mL).

+ For greater accuracy, use the smallest capacity syringe possible to measure and administer doses. However, avoid filling a syringe to its capacity.

+ When measuring two types of insulin in the same syringe, short-acting insulin is always drawn up in the syringe first.

+ The total volume when mixing insulins is the sum of the two insulin amounts.

+ Insulin syringes are for measuring and administering insulin only.

+ The prefilled single-dose syringe cartridge is to be used once and then discarded.

+ Syringes intended for injections should not be used to measure or administer oral medications.

+ Safety measures in accordance with local policies (and national Health and Safety regulations) should be adhered to for disposal of sharps and syringes (e.g. no resheathing of needles) and nurses should be aware of these.

References

Diabetes UK (2008) Guide to diabetes treatments. Available at: http://www.diabetes.org.uk/Guide-to-diabetes/Treatment_your_health/Treatments/Insulin/ (accessed March 2009).

Joint Formulary Committee (BNF) (2008) *British National Formulary* (55). London: British Medical Association and Royal Pharmaceutical Society of Great Britain.

National Institute for Health and Clinical Excellence (NICE) (2006) *Diabetes (type 1 and 2), Inhaled Insulin – Final Appraisal Determination*. London: National Institute for Health and Clinical Excellence. Available at: http://www.nice.org.uk/guidance/index.jsp?action=download&o=33787 (accessed March 2009).

Royal College of Nursing (RCN) (2006) *Standards for Infusion Therapy*. London: Royal College of Nursing.

Royal College of Nursing (RCN) (2007) *Advance preparation of insulin syringes for patients to administer at home: RCN guidance for community nurses*. London: Royal College of Nursing.

Smith J (2004) *Building a Safer NHS for Patients: Improving Medication Safety*. London: HMSO.

Summers K H, Szeinbach S L and Lenox S M (2004) Preference for insulin delivery systems among current insulin users and nonusers. *Clinical Therapeutics* **26**(9): 1498–505.

Zakrzewska J M, Greenwood I and Jackson J (2001) Introducing safety syringes into a UK Dental school – a controlled study. *British Dental Journal* **190**(2): 88–92.

Case study 6.1

On your surgical ward a 55–year-old woman with a medical history of obesity, hypertension, hyperlipidaemia and diabetes mellitus is admitted complaining of anorexia, nausea, vomiting, fever, chills and severe sharp right upper quadrant abdominal pain that radiates to her back and right shoulder. She states that her pain is 9 (on a 0–10 visual analogue pain scale). Her observations are: T 37.8 °C, BP 148/94 mmHg; P 104 beats per minute; R 24 per minute. Her diagnosis eventually reveals she has gallstones and she is to have a percutaneous cholecystectomy (removal of gall bladder).

In order to prepare for the surgical procedure, a number of interventions are planned. These pre-operative preparations include:

+ Ascertaining last food and fluid intake and for no further food or fluids orally
+ Recording of her observations initially 4 hourly to increase to more frequently if her temperature or blood pressure or pulse recordings change
+ Pethidine 75 mg IM immediately (stat) for pain
+ IV fluids: glucose-saline 125 mL/h
+ Insert a NG (nasogastric) tube if vomiting is severe and persistent
+ Pre-op medication: Phenergan (promethazine) 25 mg IM 30 minutes before surgery
+ Cefuroxime 1.5 g IV 30 minutes before surgery

Post-Operative Plan:

+ No food or fluids orally until advised this is safe
+ Recording of her observations frequently – the regularity determined by how they stabilise (may be 4 hourly or more frequently)
+ IV fluids: glucose-saline-saline 125 mL/h
+ Prochlorperazine 12.5 mg IM 4 hourly prn for nausea
+ Pethidine 75 mg 3 hourly if needed and cyclizine 10 mg IM 4 hourly as needed for pain and nausea
+ Meropenem 1 g IV every eight hours

1. The label on the pethidine vial for the stat dose reads 100 mg/mL.

   (a) Draw a line indicating the measurement on each of the following syringes below.

   (b) Which syringe will most accurately measure this dose?

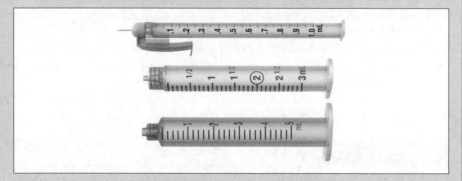

2. Calculate the pre-operative dose of the promethazine. Promethazine is available in 25 mg/mL vials.

   (a) How many millilitres of promethazine will you prepare?

   (b) Draw a line on the appropriate syringe below indicating the dose of the drug that you will administer.

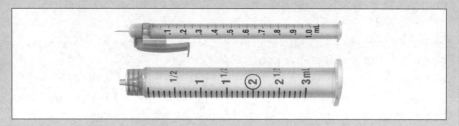

3. The label on the cefuroxime vial states: 'add 9 mL of diluent to the 1.5 g vial.' Draw a line on the appropriate syringe below indicating the amount of diluent you will add to the vial.

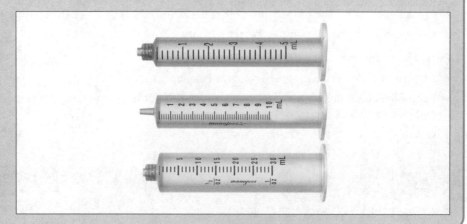

4. The patient is complaining of nausea. The Prochlorperazine vial is labelled 12.5 mg/mL. Draw a line on the syringe below indicating the dose of Prochlorperazine.

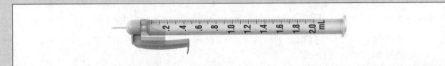

5. The patient is complaining of severe incisional pain of 10 (on a 0–10 pain scale) and has had no pain medication since her surgery. Calculate the dose of Pethidine. The Pethidine is available as 100 mg/mL.

   (a) How many millilitres of Pethidine do you need?

   (b) Indicate on the appropriate syringe below the number of millilitres you will administer.

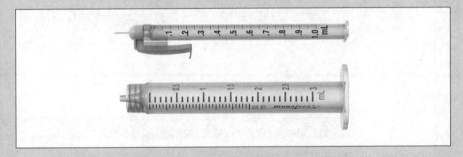

6. The label on the Meropenem states 50 mg/mL.

   (a) How many mL will you need?

   (b) Draw a line on the appropriate syringe below indicating the dose of Meropenem.

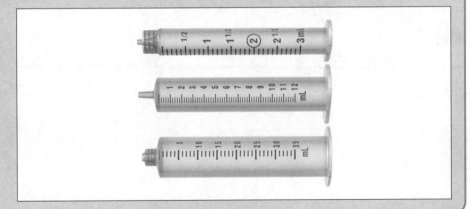

7. The patient has progressed and can now eat a normal diet and is prescribed Insulatard 13 units and Humulin S 6 units subcutaneous 30 minutes before eating breakfast, and Insulatard 5 units and Humulin S 5 units subcutaneous 30 minutes before eating dinner.

(a) How many units will the patient receive before breakfast?

(b) Indicate on the appropriate syringe below the number of units of each insulin required before breakfast.

(c) What are the advantages of using a mixed insulin such as Humulin M3 instead of the other insulins?

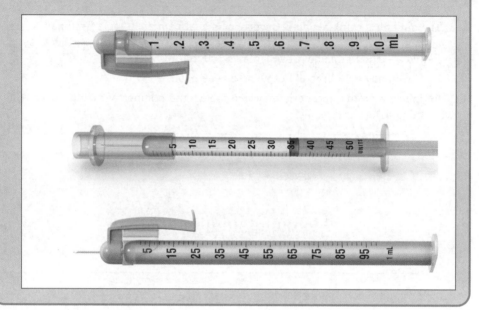

Reflection

Think back to a situation when you learned a new skill – how did you prepare to attempt this skill and how long before you became quite confident and then competent?

Reflecting on injection techniques and calculations for injections is the same as learning a new skill. List your concerns and identify how you can prepare to address these concerns and so gain confidence and competence:

1. _____

2. _____

3. _____

4. _____

5. _____

How will you know when you have improved? Make it measurable and specific!

_____

Practice sets

The answers to *Try these for practice* and *Exercises* appear in Appendix A at the end of the book.

Try these for practice

Test your comprehension after reading the chapter.

In Problems 1 to 4, identify the type of syringe shown in the figure. Place an arrow at the appropriate level of measurement on the syringe for the volume given.

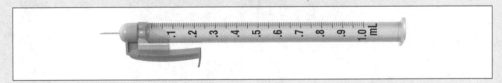

1. _____ syringe; 0.72 mL

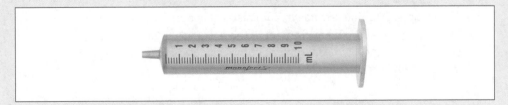

2. _____ syringe; 6.8 mL

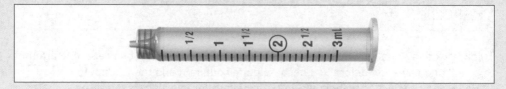

3. _____ syringe; 2.8 mL

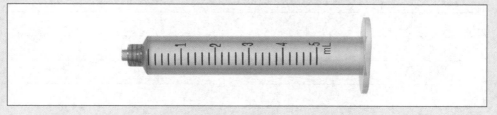

4. _____ syringe; 4.4 mL

5. The prescriber ordered 34 units of Actrapid insulin and 18 units of Insulatard subcutaneously 30 minutes before breakfast. Read the labels and do the following:

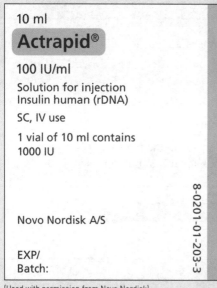

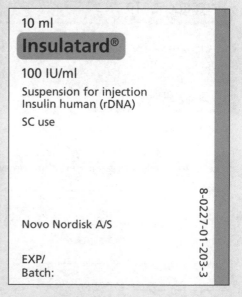

(Used with permission from Novo Nordisk)

(a) Select the appropriate syringe to administer this dose in one injection.
(b) Place an arrow at the measurement of the Actrapid insulin.
(c) Place an arrow at the measurement of the Insulatard insulin.
(d) Determine how many units the patient will receive.

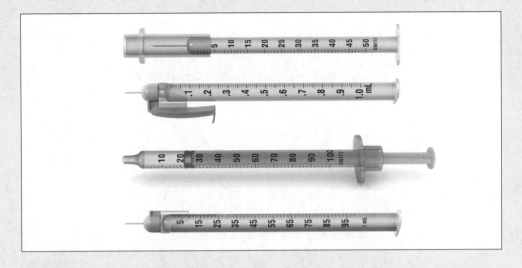

Exercises

Reinforce your understanding in class or at home.

In Exercises 1 to 10, identify the type of syringe shown in the figure. Then, for each quantity, place an arrow at the appropriate level of measurement on the syringe.

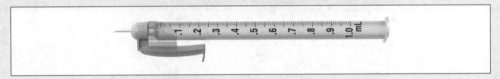

1. _____ syringe; 0.62 mL

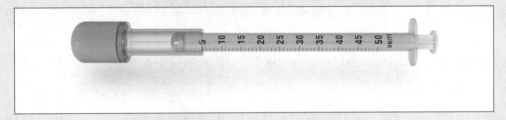

2. _____ syringe; 28 units

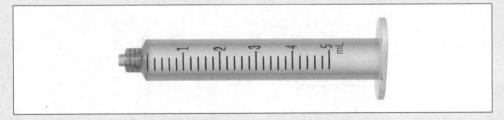

3. _____ syringe; 3.6 mL

143

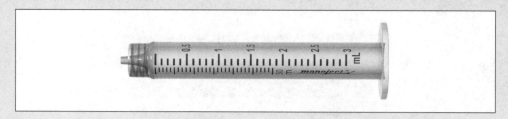

4. _____ syringe; 1.4 mL

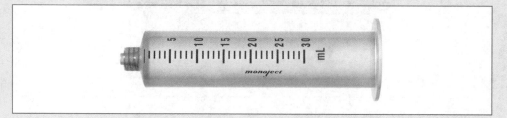

5. _____ syringe; 13 mL

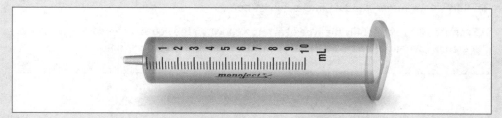

6. _____ syringe; 9.6 mL

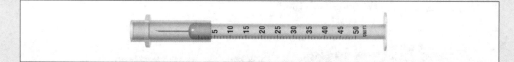

7. _____ syringe; 32 units

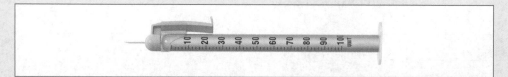

8. _____ syringe; 56 units

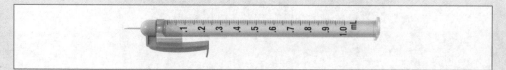

9. _____ syringe; 0.37 mL

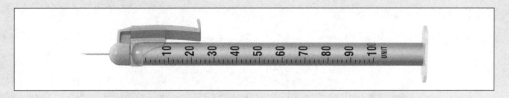

10. _____ syringe; 51 units

In Exercises 11 to 14, read the order, use the appropriate label in Figure 6.25, calculate the dosage if necessary and place an arrow at the appropriate level of measurement on the syringe.

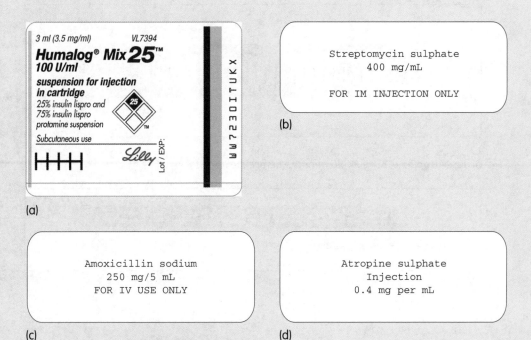

3 ml (3.5 mg/ml)   VL7394

Humalog® Mix 25™
100 U/ml

suspension for injection
in cartridge
25% insulin lispro and
75% insulin lispro
protamine suspension

Subcutaneous use

Lilly

Lot / EXP:

XXKUTIOEZ7WE

(a)

Streptomycin sulphate
400 mg/mL

FOR IM INJECTION ONLY

(b)

Amoxicillin sodium
250 mg/5 mL
FOR IV USE ONLY

(c)

Atropine sulphate
Injection
0.4 mg per mL

(d)

Figure 6.25 Drug labels for Exercises 11–14

((a) © Eli Lilly and Company. All rights reserved. Used with permission. HUMALOG® is a registered trademark of Eli Lilly and Company)

11. Prescription is for *give 26 units of Humalog 75/25 subcutaneously, 30 minutes before food (breakfast time)*.

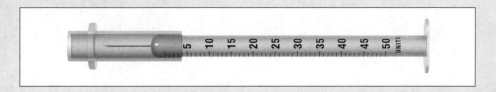

12. Prescription is for *streptomycin 600 mg IM daily*.

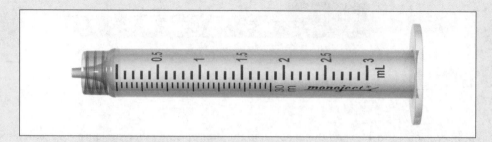

13. Prescription: *Amoxicillin 200 mg 6 hourly by IV infusion*.

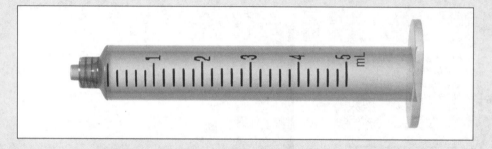

14. Order: *Atropine 0.2 mg IM 30 minutes before surgery*.

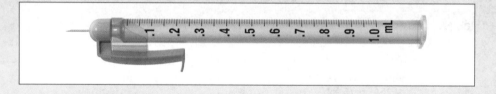

Chapter 7

Solutions and drug strengths or concentrations

Learning outcomes

After completing this chapter, you will be able to

1. Describe the strength of a solution both as a ratio and as a percentage.
2. Explain the concept of ratio in drug strength (1 in . . .).
3. Understand the concept of molar solutions.
4. Be familiar with drugs measured in units.
5. Determine the amount of drug in solutions.

In this chapter you will learn about solutions. Although solutions are generally prepared by the pharmacist, nurses and healthcare practitioners should understand the concepts involved.

Drugs are manufactured in both pure and diluted forms. A pure drug contains only the drug and nothing else. A drug is frequently diluted by dissolving a quantity of pure drug in a liquid to form a solution. The pure drug (either dry or liquid) is called the **solute**. The liquid added to the pure drug to form the solution is called the **solvent** or **diluent**. The solvents most commonly used are sterile water and normal saline solution (0.9% NaCl).

Diagnostic questions

Before commencing this chapter try the following questions to prepare you for the content and which sections to focus on. Compare your answers with those in Appendix A.

1. How many grams of glucose are there in 100 mL of a 5% glucose solution?
2. What is the other name for 'normal saline' solution?
3. A patient is to have an intravenous solution with 20 mmol of potassium. Does millimoles (mmol) refers to the weight, colour or type of potassium used in the solution?
4. A 1 in 1000 solution is stronger (more concentrated) than a 1 in 100 solution. True or False?
5. Drugs can be measured as 'units' as well as traditional weights like grams and milligrams. True or False?

Determining the strength of a medication

The variety of drug concentrations you will come across will vary and will take a range of forms, and they may be described as a drug in a particular medium, that is, drugs mixed or dissolved in a liquid medium (weight in volume or w/v), a solid mixed with another solid such as a cream or ointment (weight in weight or w/w) and finally a liquid mixed or diluted with another liquid (volume in volume or v/v). This simply means a given amount mixed or dissolved in 100 parts of the other medium. This can be abbreviated as:

w/v = grams mixed or dissolved in 100 mL of liquid

w/w = number of grams mixed with 100 g of solid

v/v = number of mLs mixed with 100 mL of liquid

The strength of a solution can also be stated as a **ratio** or a **percentage**.

+ The ratio 1:2 (read this as '1 to 2') means that there is 1 part of the drug in 2 parts of solution. This solution is also referred to as a $\frac{1}{2}$ strength solution or a 50% solution.

+ The ratio 1:10 (read this as '1 to 10') means that there is 1 part of the drug in 10 parts of solution. This solution is also referred to as a 10% solution.

+ The ratio 1:100 (read this as '1 to 100') means there is 1 part of the drug in 100 parts of the solution. This solution is referred to as a 1% solution.

+ A 5% v/v solution means that there are 5 parts of the liquid drug in 100 parts of solution.

+ A $2\frac{1}{2}$% w/v solution means that there are $2\frac{1}{2}$ parts of the solid drug in 100 parts of solution.

This has nothing to do with the volume of the container: it always refers to the basic unit of 100 – thus number of parts in 100 or *per cent.* A one litre bag or a 250 mL bag can contain 5% glucose solution, meaning the concentration of the solution is 5 parts of glucose per 100 mL irrespective of the size of the container. The size of the container is only important if you wish to find out the total amount of drug within the infusion or solution. Thus the total amount of glucose in a one litre bag will be different compared with a 250 mL bag.

Stop and think

Medications and lotions are measured in a variety of ways (weights, volumes) but can also be expressed as strengths when mixed – if a percentage, the higher the number the stronger the concentration (i.e. 50% is stronger than 20%), however, with ratios the higher the diluent number the lower the concentration (i.e. 1 in 100 is stronger than 1 in 1000).

Pure drugs in liquid form

For a pure drug that is in liquid form, the ratio 1:40 means there is 1 millilitre of pure drug in every 40 millilitres of solution. So 40 millilitres of a 1:40 acetic acid solution

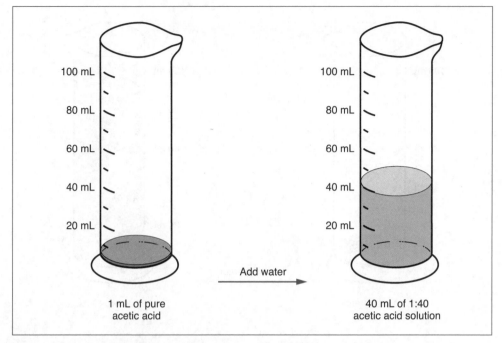

Figure 7.1 Preparing a 1:40 solution from a pure liquid drug

means that 1 millilitre of pure acetic acid is diluted with water to make a total of 40 milli-litres of solution. You would prepare this solution by placing 1 millilitre of pure acetic acid in a graduated cylinder and adding water until the level in the graduated cylinder reaches 40 millilitres (Figure 7.1).

A 5% solution means that there is 5 parts of the drug in 100 parts of solution. So you would prepare 100 mL of a 5% glucose solution by placing 5 millilitres of pure glucose in a graduated cylinder and adding water until the level in the graduated cylinder reaches 100 mL (Figure 7.2).

Example 7.1

40 mL of an iodine solution contain 14 mL of pure iodine. Express the strength of this solution both as a ratio and a percentage.

The strength of a solution may be expressed as the ratio of the *amount of pure drug in the solution to the total amount of the solution*. The amount of the *solution is always expressed in millilitres*, and because *iodine is a liquid in pure form, the amount of iodine is also expressed in millilitres*.

There are 14 mL of pure iodine in the 40 mL of the solution, so the strength of this solution, expressed as a ratio, is 14 to 40. The ratio may also be written as *14:40, 14 to 40* or, in fractional form, as $\frac{14}{40}$. This fraction could then be simplified to $\frac{7}{20}$, which is equal to 35% (i.e. 7 divided by 20 = 0.35 or 35%).

So, the strength of this iodine solution may be expressed as the ratio *7:20* or the percentage *35%*.

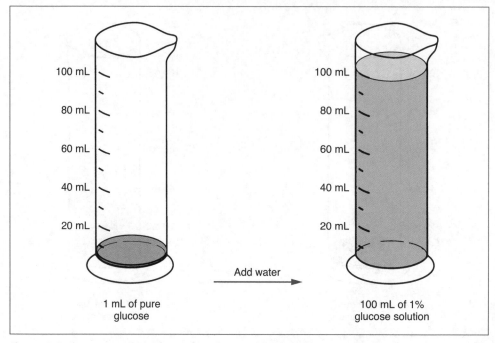

100 mL

80 mL

60 mL

40 mL

20 mL

100 mL

80 mL

60 mL

40 mL

20 mL

Add water

1 mL of pure
glucose

100 mL of 1%
glucose solution

Figure 7.2 Preparing a 1% solution from a pure liquid drug

Pure drugs in dry form

The ratio 1:20 means 1 part of the pure drug in 20 parts of solution. This is also the same as 2 parts of the pure drug in 40 parts of solution, or 3 parts in 60, or 4 parts in 80, or 5 parts in 100, and so on. When a pure drug is in dry form, the ratio 1:20 means 1 g of pure drug in every 20 mL of solution. Consider a pharmacist preparing a topical solution, such as 100 mL of a 1:20 potassium permanganate solution. This means the pharmacist takes *5 g* of pure potassium permanganate and dissolves this in water to make a total of *100 mL* of the solution. This is therefore a concentration of 1:20 which also equals a concentration of 5:100. A 1:20 solution is the same as a 5% solution because this is also the same as $\dfrac{5\ g}{100\ mL}$ (remember 5 divided by 100 = 0.05 or 5%). The final volume must equal 100 mL, not 100 mL *added* to the tablet as this would change the final volume (perhaps make it 105 mL) which would alter the concentration. See Figure 7.3.

Example 7.2

One litre of an isotonic normal saline solution contains 9000 mg of sodium chloride. Express the strength of this solution both as a ratio and as a percentage.

The strength of a solution may be expressed as the ratio of the *amount of pure drug* in the solution to the *total amount of the solution*. Since sodium chloride (NaCl) is a *solid* in pure form, the amount of NaCl (9000 mg) must be expressed in *grams* (9 g). The *amount of the solution* (1 L) must always be expressed in *millilitres* (1000 mL). Since there are 9 g of

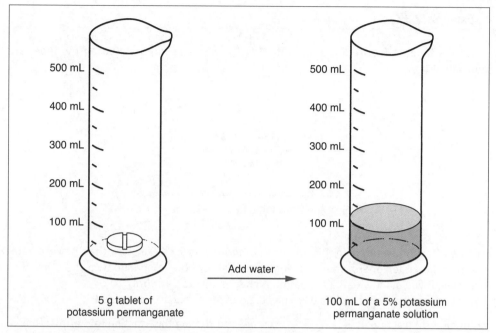

Figure 7.3 Preparation of a 5% solution from dry drug

pure NaCl in 1000 mL of the solution, the strength of this solution, expressed as a ratio, is *nine to one thousand*.

This ratio may also be written as *9 to 1000*, *9:1000* or, in fractional form, as $\frac{9}{1000}$. This fraction could be written in decimal form as 0.009 g in 1 mL. Thus in 100 mL (to make a percent = X parts in 100) is equal to 0.9%.

So, the strength of this isotonic normal saline solution may be expressed as the ratio *9:1000* or the percentage *0.9%*.

In summary:

$$
\begin{aligned}
\text{Sodium chloride (0.9\%)} &= 9 \text{ g per 1 L} \\
&= 0.9 \text{ g per 100 mL} \\
&= 900 \text{ mg per 100 mL} \\
&= 9 \text{ mg/mL} \\
&= 0.9 \text{ g/100} \\
&= 0.9\%
\end{aligned}
$$

Practice point

0.9% NaCl is widely used as an intravenous fluid for rehydration of patients in hospitals. In cases where patients need to have their sodium intake monitored, such as those with renal problems, it may be necessary to calculate the amount of sodium in IV fluids.

Example 7.3

Read the label in Figure 7.4 and verify that the two strengths stated on the label are equivalent.

Ropivacaine HCl injection
For epidural use
2 mg/mL 0.2%

Figure 7.4 Drug label for ropivacaine

The two strengths stated on this label are *2 mg/mL and 0.2%*. To show that they are equivalent, take either one of these strengths and show how to change it to the other. For example, if you start with 0.2%, you must change this to 2 mg/mL.

A solution whose strength is 0.2% has 0.2 g of pure drug (ropivacaine HCl) in 100 mL of solution. As a fraction, this is $\dfrac{0.2 \text{ g}}{100 \text{ mL}}$. You need to change this fraction to mg/mL. That is:

$$\frac{0.2 \text{ g}}{100 \text{ mL}} = \frac{? \text{ mg}}{\text{mL}}$$

To change the grams in the numerator to milligrams, use the equivalence 1 g = 1000 mg:

$$\frac{0.2 \text{ g}}{100 \text{ mL}} \times \frac{1000 \text{ mg}}{1 \text{ g}} = \frac{2 \text{ mg}}{\text{mL}}$$

So, the two strengths stated on the label, 2 mg/mL and 0.2%, are equivalent.

Consider Adrenaline (Epinephrine). This is available in 1:1000 and 1:10 000 concentration, however, you want to know which is the stronger concentration?

1:1000 = 1 g in 1000 mL

1:10 000 = 1 g in 10 000 mL

Thus 1:1000 concentration is stronger as it is less dilute – note the higher the number for the diluent the weaker the concentration.

Determining the amount of pure drug in a given amount of solution

The units of measurement for the amount of solution (volume), strength of the solution, and amount of pure drug are listed as follows:

Amount of solution: Use *millilitres*.

Strength: Always write as a fraction for calculations.

For liquids: 1:40 acetic acid solution is written as $\dfrac{1\ \text{mL}}{40\ \text{mL}}$

5% acetic acid solution is written as $\dfrac{5\ \text{mL}}{100\ \text{mL}}$

For tablets or powder: 1:20 potassium permanganate solution is written as $\dfrac{1\ \text{g}}{20\ \text{mL}}$

12% potassium permanganate solution is written as $\dfrac{12\ \text{g}}{100\ \text{mL}}$

Amount of pure drug: Use *millilitres* for liquids.

Use *grams* for tablets or powders.

In order to prepare a given amount of a solution of a given strength, you must first determine the amount of pure drug that will be in that solution. The following examples illustrate how this is done.

Example 7.4

Read the label in Figure 7.5. How many grams of dextrose (glucose) are contained in 30 mL of this solution?

```
           50% Glucose
            Injection
   25 grams (500 mg/mL)
      50 mL container
```

Figure 7.5 Drug label for 50% glucose

Given: Amount of solution: 30 mL

Strength: 50% or $\dfrac{50}{100}$, so you use $\dfrac{50\ \text{g}}{100\ \text{mL}}$

153

Find: Amount of pure drug: ? g

$$30 \text{ mL} \times \frac{50 \text{ g}}{100 \text{ mL}} = ? \text{ g}$$

$$\cancel{30 \text{ mL}} \times \frac{50 \text{ g}}{\cancel{100 \text{ mL}}} = 15 \text{ g}$$

So, *15 g* of glucose are contained in 30 mL of a 50% glucose solution.

Practice point

Diabetic patients having IV fluids may need particular attention if the fluid is 5% glucose (also called dextrose) which will have an effect on their blood sugar. If not monitored, this could lead to an overdose of glucose and serious consequences for the patient (i.e. hyperglycaemia).

Example 7.5

Read the label in Figure 7.6 and determine the number of milligrams of Lidocaine that are contained in 5 mL of this Lidocaine solution.

Lidocaine 4%
Topical anaesthetic spray
50 mL

Figure 7.6 Drug label for Lidocaine

Given: Amount of solution: 5 mL
Strength: 4%
Find: Amount of pure drug: ? mg

You want to convert the amount of the solution (5 mL) to the amount of the pure drug (? mg):

$$5 \text{ mL} = ? \text{ mg}$$

Note that Lidocaine is a powder in pure form, so the strength of the 4% solution is expressed in fraction form as $\dfrac{4\ g}{100\ mL}$. This strength can be used to find the amount of Lidocaine in grams:

$$5\ \cancel{mL} \times \frac{4\ \text{\textcircled{g}}}{100\ \cancel{mL}} = ?\ mg$$

But you want the answer in milligrams, so the equivalence 1 g = 1000 mg must also be used. This can be written in one line as follows:

$$5\ \cancel{mL} \times \frac{4\ \cancel{g}}{100\ \cancel{mL}} \times \frac{1000\ mg}{\cancel{g}} = 200\ mg$$

So, *200 mg* of Lidocaine are contained in 5 mL of a 4% Lidocaine solution.

Stop and think

There are 3 quantities associated with a solution: the strength of the solution, the amount of pure drug dissolved in the solution and the total volume of the solution. If any of 2 of these 3 quantities is known, the other quantity can be found.

Determining the amount of solution that contains a given amount of pure drug

In the previous examples, you were *given a volume of solution* of known strength and had to *find the amount of pure drug* in that solution. Now, the process will be reversed. In the following examples, you will be *given an amount of the pure drug* in a solution of known strength and have to *find the volume of that solution*.

Example 7.6

How many millilitres of a 20% magnesium sulphate solution will contain 40 g of the pure drug magnesium sulphate?

You need to determine the number of millilitres of this solution, which contains 40 g of pure drug.

Given: Amount of pure drug: 40 g
         Strength: 20%
Find: Amount of solution: ? mL

You want to convert the 40 g of pure drug to millilitres of solution:

$$40\ g = ?\ mL$$

155

You want to cancel the grams and obtain the equivalent amount in millilitres:

$$40 \text{ g} \times \frac{? \text{ mL}}{? \text{ g}} = ? \text{ mL}$$

In a 20% solution there are 20 g of magnesium sulphate per 100 mL of solution. So, the fraction is

$$\frac{100 \text{ mL}}{20 \text{ g}}$$

$$\overset{2}{40 \text{ g}} \times \frac{100 \text{ mL}}{\underset{1}{20 \text{ g}}} = 200 \text{ mL}$$

So, *200 mL* of a 20% magnesium sulphate solution contains 40 g of magnesium sulphate.

Check your answer – with this example you can see a pattern: if it is 20% strength, this means 20 g in 100 mL; thus for 40 g it would be 200 mL. Always check back to ensure you have the correct answer.

Molar solutions and molarity

Some older pharmacology textbooks and overseas texts refer to milliequivalents for drugs or even biochemical values. This is not part of the SI system and thus not accepted for daily use. Instead of this, **molarity** is the accepted system which uses units based on moles, millimoles and, on occasion, micromoles. Molarity is another way of expressing the strength or concentration of a solution or medicine. It is often also used in expressing the concentration of biochemical substances such as potassium or glucose monitored in the blood of patients or clients. In clinical practice, it is useful to have a basic under-standing of molarity and molar solutions, not least for biochemical data but also for administration of medicinal products. One must refer to basic chemistry to understand the fundamental principles; however, for a more in-depth explanation do delve into a good chemistry textbook.

All elements are made up of atoms, and these are too small to be counted or weighed individually. The mole is a method used by chemists to make counting atoms easier by weighing them. Each individual atom has its own unique **atomic weight** (sometimes called mass). Atoms combine to form molecules, e.g. an atom of sodium (Na) can com-bine with chloride (Cl) to form sodium chloride (NaCl). Thus if each atom has its own **atomic weight** then atoms combined (molecules) have a combined weight called the **molecular weight**. These weights are outlined in various chemistry texts; only a few are included here:

Sodium (Na)	atomic weight = 23
Potassium (K)	atomic weight = 39
Calcium (Ca)	atomic weight = 40
Chloride (Cl)	atomic weight = 35.4
Sodium chloride (NaCl)	molecular weight (23 + 35.4) = 58.4
Potassium chloride (KCl)	molecular weight (39 + 35.4) = 74.4

A **mole** represents the weight in grams of the atom or molecule the same as the relative molecular or atomic weight. For example the molecular weight of sodium chloride is 58.4, thus 1 mole is 58.4 g.

+ A molar solution contains 1 mole in 1 litre of solvent. Thus a 1 molar solution of sodium chloride contains 58.4 g of sodium chloride in 1 litre of solvent.
+ A millimolar solution is the molar solution divided by 1000.
+ In percentage terms, 58.4 g of sodium chloride in 1 litre = $58.4/1000 \times 100 = 5.84\%$ w/v.

Use of moles and millimoles

Nurses generally are not required to calculate moles or millimoles or make up solutions using these fundamental chemistry principles. However, they should be familiar with the terms as they may be administering drugs or intravenous infusion solutions expressed as moles or millimoles/L. At times solid drugs may be expressed as millimolar concentration, e.g. electrolyte replacement tablets (potassium, etc.). In addition, blood biochemistry results are identified this way (e.g. blood glucose mmol/L) and consequent administration of prescribed variable dose drug therapy.

Stop and think

> Moles are just another way of expressing a weight and concentration of a solution. Look at blood test results for a patient: sodium, bicarbonate and other electrolytes are all measured in mmol/L; that is, a weight (mmol) in a volume (litre of blood).

Drugs measured in units

For certain drugs, due to the variable purity from the animal or biochemical sources, the standard measurement used is the unit rather than the familiar weights and volumes. These include drugs such as **heparin** and **insulin**. The abbreviation of the term unit and the various symbols used have led to confusion and drug errors (Smith 2004). Thus, according to the BNF (2008) and Smith (2004) it is imperative and also good practice that the term *unit* must be written in full to avoid confusion between prescriber and whoever is administering the drug.

There are two main types of heparin available for patient use: standard heparin and low molecular weight heparin. Additionally, these are available either as prefilled syringes or in vials to be drawn up for use. Thus, in the case of the latter reading the labels and calculation of doses are important. Heparin is available in a variety of strengths expressed as units per mL. These include:

1000 units/mL
5000 units/mL
10 000 units/mL
25 000 units/mL

The initial dose may be different from the maintenance dose and caution is recommended with checking the heparin type, dosage regime and calculations accordingly (see Chapter 8).

Example 7.7

A patient is prescribed an immediate dose of heparin 4000 units IV followed by a continuous infusion of heparin 25 000 units IV over 24 hours. Another patient on the ward is prescribed heparin 10 000 units subcutaneously 12 hourly. What is the main difference between the two prescriptions? What are the consequences if you give 25 000 units subcutaneously?

There are two main differences – the dosage and the route. The main consequence of giving 25 000 units subcutaneously is an excessive dose (in this instance prolonged bleeding). This would be a serious drug error and the nurse or whoever gave the medication is responsible (NMC 2008).

Summary

In this chapter, you learned that there are drugs which are measured in units (heparin and insulin), although the units have no equivalencies among differing drugs. These need to be accepted for each drug used and care taken when reading labels and prescription charts. Also that there are 3 quantities associated with a solution: the strength of the solution, the amount of pure drug dissolved in the solution and the total volume of the solution. If any 2 of these 3 quantities is known, the other quantity can be found.

+ The strength of a solution may be expressed as a ratio or as a percentage.

+ The strength of a solution is the ratio of the amount of pure drug dissolved in the solution to the total volume of the solution.

+ The volume of the solution should be expressed in millilitres.

+ The amount of pure drug dissolved in the solution should be expressed in millilitres if the drug, in its pure form, is a liquid.

+ The amount of pure drug dissolved in the solution should be expressed in grams if the drug, in its pure form, is a solid.

+ A $\frac{1}{2}$ strength solution is a 50% solution, and should not be confused with a $\frac{1}{2}$% solution.

+ To determine the amount of drug in a given amount of solution of known strength, start with the given amount of solution.

+ To determine the amount of solution of known strength containing a given amount of drug, start with the given amount of drug.

References

Joint Formulary Committee (BNF) (2008) *British National Formulary 55*. London: British Medical Association and Royal Pharmaceutical Society of Great Britain.

Nursing and Midwifery Council (NMC) (2008) *Standards for Medicines Management*. London: Nursing and Midwifery Council.

Smith J (2004) *Building a Safer NHS for Patients: Improving Medication Safety*. London: HMSO.

Case study 7.1

A 75-year-old woman is admitted to a general medical ward following a successful mitral valve replacement surgery. This lady has a past medical history of osteoarthritis, hypertension, atrial fibrillation and Type I (insulin-dependent) diabetes mellitus. On assessment it appears she has a 3 cm wound on the right heel. Prior to surgery she was an independent lady who cared for herself with only support of meals on wheels until the last year when she tired easily. She is overweight and realises she does need to lose weight if her osteoarthritis and diabetes are to improve. She is alert and oriented to person, place, time and recent memory. She rates her pain level as 6 on a 0–10 visual analogue scale. Her observations are: T 37.5 °C; P 68/min; R 18/min; B/P 124/76 mmHg.

On admission her medications are:

+ Dipyridamole (Persantin) 75 mg PO, q.d.s.
+ Amiodarone hydrochloride (Cordarone) 400 mg PO daily
+ Diltiazem SR (Dilzem SR) 180 mg PO daily
+ Nabumetone (Relifex) 1000 mg PO daily
+ Potassium chloride (KCl) oral solution 20 mmol PO b.i.d.
+ Multi-vitamin 1 tab PO daily
+ Paracetamol 1 g PO 4 hourly prn if temperature above 38 °C
+ Humulin S insulin 10 units and Humulin I insulin 38 units subcutaneous 30 min before breakfast
+ Humulin S insulin 10 units and Humulin I insulin 30 units 30 min before dinner
+ Pneumoccoccal vaccine (Pneumovax II) 0.5 mL IM × 1 dose
+ Cleanse right heel with normal saline solution (0.9% NaCl) and apply a dry dressing daily
+ 1800 calorie and maximum 2 g sodium diet

Refer to the labels in Figure 7.7 when necessary to answer the following questions:

1. The Pneumovax II vial contains 2.5 mL. Choose the appropriate syringe from those below and place an arrow at the dose.
2. Diltiazem (Dilzem SR) is available in 60 mg and 120 mg tablets. Which strength will you use and how many tablets for the daily dose?
3. The potassium chloride (KCL) solution label reads 40 mmol/15 mL. How many millilitres will you administer?

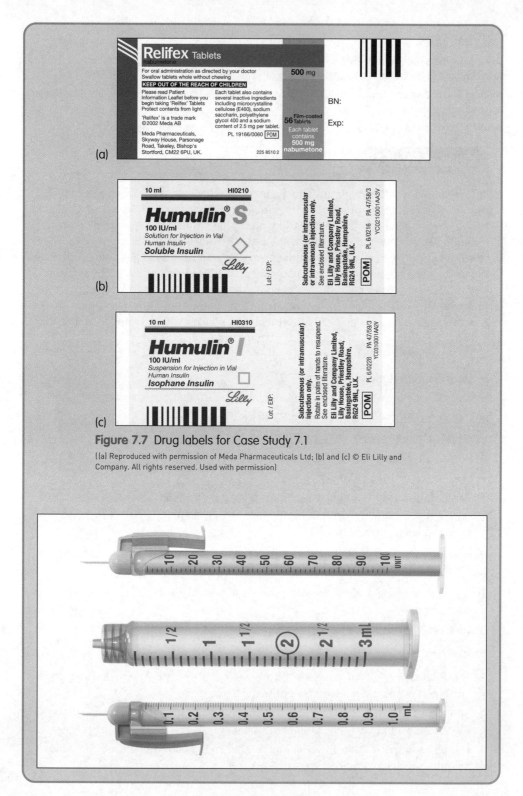

Figure 7.7 Drug labels for Case Study 7.1

((a) Reproduced with permission of Meda Pharmaceuticals Ltd; (b) and (c) © Eli Lilly and Company. All rights reserved. Used with permission)

4. The dipyridamole (Persantin) is available in 25, 50 and 75 mg tablets. Which strength tablets will you administer and how many?

5. How many tablets of nabumetone (Relifex) will you administer?

6. Describe how you will measure the morning insulin. Select the appropriate syringe from those below and mark the dose of Humulin S and Humulin I.

7. How many grams of sodium chloride (NaCl) are in 1 L of the saline solution?

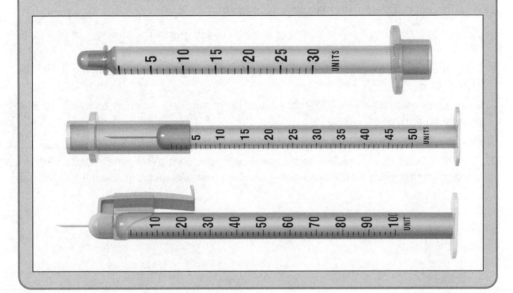

Practice sets

The answers to *Try these for practice* and *Exercises* appear in Appendix A at the end of the book.

Try these for practice

Test your comprehension after reading the chapter.

1. 320 mL of a solution contain 80 mg of a pure drug. Express the strength of this solution as a percent. _____

2. How would you prepare 1 L of a 10% solution from tablets each containing 5 g of the pure drug? _____

3. How many millilitres of a 25% potassium permanganate solution contains 20 g of potassium permanganate? _____

4. How would you prepare 200 mL of a 5% solution from a 20% stock solution? _____

5. Read the label in Figure 7.8 and show how you would determine that two of the strengths mentioned on the label are equivalent (use 500 mcg/2 mL and 0.5 mg/2mL). _____

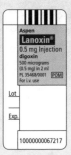

Figure 7.8 Drug label for Lanoxin

(Reproduced with permission from Aspen Pharmacare)

Exercises

Reinforce your understanding in class or at home.

1. 750 mL of a solution contain 15 mL of a pure drug. Express the strength of this solution both as a ratio and as a percentage.

2. Two litres of a solution contain 60 g of a pure drug. Express the strength of this solution both as a ratio and as a percentage.

3. How much sodium chloride is contained in 300 mL of a 0.9% sodium chloride hydrochloride?

4. Read the label in Figure 7.9 and determine the number of milligrams of hydroxyzine hydrochloride that are contained in the vial.

```
Hydroxyzine hydrochloride
     Syrup 10 mg/mL
```

Figure 7.9 Drug label for hydroxyzine

5. How many millilitres of hydroxyzine (see Figure 7.9) contain 20 mg of hydroxyzine hydrochloride?

6. How many millilitres of a 6% solution contain 18 g of the pure drug?

7. Read the label in Figure 7.10. How many millilitres of this solution contain 300 mg of Lidocaine HCl?

```
       Lidocaine 4%
Topical anaesthetic spray
        50 mL
```

Figure 7.10 Drug label for Xylocaine

8. If 600 mL of a solution contain 120 mL of a pure drug, express the strength of this solution both as a ratio and as a percentage.

9. If 1 L of a solution contains 2000 mg of a pure drug, express the strength of this solution both as a ratio and as a percentage.

```
Metoprolol tartrate
injection for IV use
    5 mg/5 mL
  (5 mL ampoule)
```

Figure 7.11 Drug label for metoprolol

10. Read the label in Figure 7.11 and determine the number of millilitres that would contain 35 mg of pure metoprolol tartrate.

11. A drug label states the strength of the solution is 10 mg/mL or 1%. Verify that the two stated strengths are equivalent.

12. Read the label in Figure 7.11 and determine how many milligrams of metoprolol tartrate are contained in 12 mL.

Chapter 8

Parenteral medications

Learning outcomes

After completing this chapter, you will be able to

1. Calculate doses for parenteral medications in liquid form.

2. Describe how to reconstitute medications in powder form.

3. Calculate doses of parenteral medications measured in units.

This chapter introduces you to the calculations you will use to prepare and administer parenteral medications safely. Chapter 2 discussed the most common parenteral sites: intramuscular (IM), subcutaneous (subcut), intravenous (IV) and intradermal (ID). This chapter will focus on calculations for administering medications via the subcutaneous and intramuscular routes.

Diagnostic questions

Before commencing this chapter do try the following questions. Compare your answers with those in Appendix A. Focus on areas you feel need attention and try to relate the exercises in the chapter to your own clinical practice.

1. A medication which is stated on the package as 10 mg/10 mL is the same as 1 mg/mL. True or False?

2. You need to prepare 375 mcg of a drug and it is available as 500 mcg in 5 mL. On estimation, before calculation, do you need more or less than 3 mL?

3. To reconstitute a powder drug, the liquid you add (the diluent) is always water for injection. True or False?

4. After reconstituting a drug there may be an additional volume, e.g. adding 2.5 mL of diluent may lead to a total final volume of 3 mL. Why is this?

5. A cluttered and untidy clinical preparation room is one factor in drug errors. Fact or Fiction?

Parenteral medications

Parenteral medications are those that are injected into the body by various routes. Drugs for parenteral medications may be packaged in a variety of forms, including ampoules, vials and prefilled cartridges or syringes. Prefilled cartridges and syringes were discussed in Chapter 6.

An **ampoule** is a glass container that holds a single dose of medication. It has a narrowed neck that is designed to snap open. The medication is aspirated into a syringe by gently pulling back on the plunger, which creates a negative pressure and allows the liquid to be pulled into the syringe (Figure 8.1).

A **vial** is a glass or plastic container that has a rubber stopper on the top. This stopper is covered with a lid that maintains the sterility of the stopper until the vial is used for the first time. Multidose vials contain more than one dose of a medication. Single-dose vials contain a single dose of medication, and many drugs are now prepared in this format to reduce the chance of error. The medication in a vial may be in liquid or powdered form (Figure 8.2).

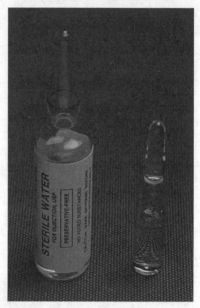

Figure 8.1 Ampoules

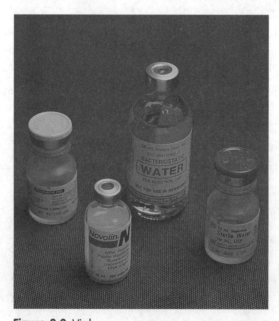

Figure 8.2 Vials

Practice point

Single-dose ampoules and vials may contain a little more drug than indicated on the label. Therefore, if the prescription is for the exact amount of medication stated on the label, it is very important to carefully measure the amount of medication to be withdrawn. If in doubt check the instructions with the drug or with the pharmacy. Before a fluid can be extracted from a vial, that same volume of air or diluent must first be injected into the vial.

Parenteral medications supplied as liquids

When parenteral medications are in liquid form, you must calculate the volume of the solution that contains the prescribed amount of the medication. You also need to know the strength of the solution.

Example 8.1

The prescriber orders a drug 600 mg IM stat and 400 mg IM 4 hourly prn. The label on the vial indicates 80 mg/mL and the total volume in the vial is 10 mL. Calculate the number of millilitres of this drug you will administer to the patient immediately (stat).

Begin by determining how many millilitres of the liquid in the vial contain the prescribed quantity of the medication (600 mg – the question asks for the stat dose!). That is, you want to convert 600 mg to an equivalent in millilitres.

$$600 \text{ mg} = ? \text{ mL}$$

You cancel the milligrams and obtain the equivalent quantity in millilitres:

$$600 \text{ mg} \times \frac{? \text{ mL}}{? \text{ mg}} = ? \text{ mL}$$

The label reads 80 mg per millilitre, which means the solution strength is 80 mg/1 mL. Thus, when you begin your estimation to see approximately how much you will need to prepare, it will be more than 1 mL (80 mg) or 5 mL (400 mg) and less than 10 mL (800 mg) so between 5 and 10 mL approximately. So, the unit fraction is $\frac{1 \text{ mL}}{80 \text{ mg}}$:

$$600 \text{ mg} \times \frac{1 \text{ mL}}{80 \text{ mg}} = \frac{60 \text{ mL}}{8} = 7.5 \text{ mL}$$

So, you would administer *7.5 mL* to the patient.

Check your answer using the other formula (amount wanted/amount available × volume of available amount) it will work with parenteral as well as oral medications. This is an additional check, but using the above will help ensure you understand which units of measurement are being used and which make the answer:

Amount wanted: 600 mg

Amount available: 80 mg

Volume: 1 mL

So, 600 mg/80 mg × 1 mL = 7.5 mL – the same!!

Example 8.2

The prescriber orders *prochlorperazine (Stemetil) 7 mg IM 4 hourly prn*. The label on the prochlorperazine states 5 mg/mL and it is a 10 mL multidose vial. Calculate how many millilitres of this anti-emetic you will administer to the patient.

Begin by determining how many millilitres of the liquid in the vial contain the prescribed quantity of the medication. That is, you want to convert 7 mg to an equivalent in millilitres:

$$7 \text{ mg} = ? \text{ mL}$$

You cancel the milligrams and obtain the equivalent quantity in millilitres.

Next, estimate approximately what volume would sound correct. You want 7 mg, the label states 5 mg/mL; thus you want more than 1 mL but less than 2 mL (10 mg/2 mL). Thus:

$$7 \text{ mg} \times \frac{? \text{ mL}}{? \text{ mg}} = ? \text{ mL}$$

The label reads 5 mg per millilitre. So, the unit fraction is $\dfrac{1 \text{ mL}}{5 \text{ mg}}$:

$$7 \text{ mg} \times \frac{1 \text{ mL}}{5 \text{ mg}} = 1.4 \text{ mL}$$

So, you would administer *1.4 mL* to the patient. Check this answer another way to ensure it is correct.

Example 8.3

A patient is prescribed *digoxin (Lanoxin) 600 mcg IV bolus (push) stat.* Read the label in Figure 8.3 and determine how many millilitres of this anti-arrhythmic cardiac glycoside you will prepare.

Begin by determining how many millilitres of the solution in the vial contain the prescribed quantity of the medication. That is, you want to convert 600 mcg to an equivalent in millilitres:

$$600 \text{ mcg} = ? \text{ mL}$$

Next, estimate what approximate volume would sound correct – the label indicates 250 mcg in 1 mL or 500 mcg in 2 mL – so it is more than 2 mL, but 3 mL would be 750 mcg so it is not as much as

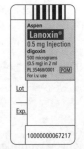

Figure 8.3 Drug label for Lanoxin

(Reproduced with permission from Aspen Pharmacare)

3 mL, so it is between 2 and 3 mL. You cancel the micrograms and obtain the equivalent quantity in millilitres:

$$600 \text{ mcg} \times \frac{? \text{ mL}}{? \text{ mcg}} = ? \text{ mL}$$

The label indicates that there are 250 mcg per millilitre. So, the unit fraction is $\dfrac{1 \text{ mL}}{250 \text{ mcg}}$:

$$\overset{12}{\cancel{600 \text{ mcg}}} \times \frac{1 \text{ mL}}{\underset{5}{\cancel{250 \text{ mcg}}}} = \frac{12 \text{ mL}}{5} = 2.4 \text{ mL}$$

So, you would give the patient 2.4 mL as an immediate IV injection.

___

Example 8.4

The prescriber orders an anti-emetic drug for a patient. The dose indicated is 200 mg IM stat. You have a 20 mL multidose vial, and the label indicates that the strength is 100 mg/mL. How many millilitres of this anti-emetic drug will you prepare?

The first step is estimation from the information available: you want to prepare 200 mg; the vial indicates 100 mg/mL so it is between 1 and 2 mL.

Next, determine how many millilitres of the solution in the vial contain the prescribed quantity of the medication. That is, you want to convert 200 mg to an equivalent in millilitres:

$$200 \text{ mg} = ? \text{ mL}$$

You cancel the milligrams and obtain the equivalent quantity in millilitres:

$$200 \text{ mg} \times \frac{? \text{ mL}}{? \text{ mg}} = ? \text{ mL}$$

The label indicates that there are 100 mg per millilitre. So, the unit fraction is $\dfrac{1 \text{ mL}}{100 \text{ mg}}$:

$$\cancel{200 \text{ mg}} \times \frac{1 \text{ mL}}{\cancel{100 \text{ mg}}} = 2 \text{ mL}$$

So, you would give the patient 2 mL.

___

Parenteral medications supplied in powdered form

Some parenteral medications are unstable when stored in liquid form, so they are packaged in powdered form. Before they can be administered, the powder in the vial must be diluted with a liquid (*diluent*). This process is referred to as **reconstitution**. Drugs and medications in this form need to be given as soon as they are reconstituted due to their limited stability (NPSA 2007).

Sterile water and 0.9% sodium chloride (normal saline) are the most commonly used *diluents*. Both the type and amount of diluent to be used must be determined when reconstituting parenteral medications. This information is found on the medication label or summary of product characteristics (SPC) leaflet. Because many reconstituted parenteral medications can be administered either intramuscularly or intravenously, it is essential to verify the route ordered **before** reconstituting the medication. This may have implications not only for the volume of diluent used but also for the eventual product to be administered to the patient. You should have all equipment ready to reconstitute the drug which is to be administered; a cluttered clinical utility room or preparation area has been identified as a key component in drug errors and should be minimised at all times (Smith 2004). Drugs dissolve completely in the diluent. Some drugs do not add any volume to the amount of diluent added, while other drugs increase the amount of total volume. This increase in volume is called the **displacement factor**. For example, directions for a 1 g powdered medication may state to add 2 mL of diluent to provide an approximate volume of 2.5 mL. When the 2 mL of diluent is added, the 1 g of powdered drug displaces an additional 0.5 mL for a total volume of 2.5 mL. That means that the dry power drug has a weight of its own and when dissolved in the diluent made up the extra 0.5 mL volume. The available strength after reconstitution is 400 mg/mL. If there are no directions for reconstitution on the label or package leaflet, consult appropriate resources such as the British National Formulary (BNF), Electronic Medicines Compendium (EMC) or the pharmacist.

Some medications are manufactured and packaged with the diluent; this makes it clearer which and how much diluent is to be used. There may also be products which are manufactured with automatic mixing devices. However, these may be expensive and more non-proprietary brands may be preferred at a particular institution. If supplied as a 'kit' this does not mean you should be complacent about checking the diluent, expiration of both medication and diluent, using aseptic processes, and still checking the final medication product for clarity prior to administration. See Figure 8.4.

Stop and think

When mixing up medications it may be that the powdered drug when reconstituted is a larger volume than the diluent added. For example, the label states that for drug X when 2.5 mL of diluent is added, the resulting solution has an approximate volume of 3 mL yielding a strength of 330 mg/mL. This is due to the displacement factor of 0.5 mL, which adds 0.5 mL to the total volume. This is only an issue if you are drawing up doses less than the final amount, e.g. 300 mg from a vial reconstituted yielding a final amount of 330 mg/mL.

Example 8.5

The prescriber orders an antibiotic medication 265 mg IM 8 hourly. The directions on the label state: 'For IM use, add 2.5 mL of sterile water for injection and shake well. The resulting solution has an approximate volume of 3 mL yielding a strength of 330 mg/mL.' Describe how you would prepare this antibiotic. How many millilitres will you administer to the patient?

Drug is IMIPENEM (Primaxin 500 mg for IV use)

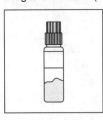

Step 1 EXAMINE

Examine the vial for any foreign material in the powder and make sure the tamper-evident seal between the cap and the vial is intact.

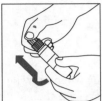

Step 2 REMOVE CAP

Remove the cap by first twisting it and pulling it up to break the tamper-evident seal.

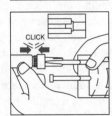

Step 3 CONNECT

Insert the needle into the infusion-bag connector. *Push* the needle-holder and vial together until they click into place.

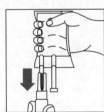

Step 4 MIX

Hold the vial in an upright position. *Squeeze* the infusion bag several times to transfer the diluent into the vial. Shake the vial to reconstitute the substance.

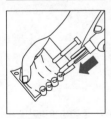

Step 5 TRANSFER

Now reverse the connected IV assembly, holding the vial upside down. Squeeze the infusion bag several times. This will create an over-pressure in the vial, allowing the contents of the vial to be transferred back into the infusion bag. Repeat steps 4 and 5 until the vial is completely empty.

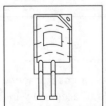

Step 6 IDENTIFY

Fill out the peel-off label on the vial and *affix* it to the infusion bag for proper identification

Figure 8.4 Mix-o-Vial of Imipenem

(From Merck Sharp & Dohme Ltd, reproduced with permission)

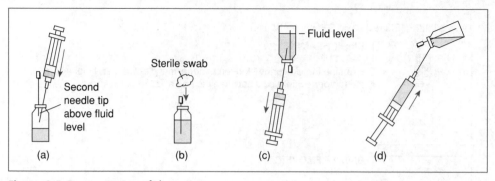

Figure 8.5 Reconstitution of drug

(Adapted from Dougherty and Lister (eds) (2008))

First, it is important to minimise environmental exposure of the drug when drawing up. Lister (2008: 207) suggests a method as outlined in Figure 8.5. To prepare the solution, insert a second needle into the vial to allow air to escape when adding the diluent for injection. Draw up 2.5 mL of sterile water. Then add the 2.5 mL of sterile water to the vial and shake well. When shaking the vial to dissolve the powder, push in the second needle up to the Luer connection and cover with a sterile swab. To draw up the reconstituted medication solution insert the syringe needle and invert the vial. The second needle should be above the fluid, then withdraw the medication solution to the desired amount as indicated in the marks of the syringe. It is important to remove air from the syringe by injecting back into the vial and not spraying it into the atmosphere. Should there be other forms of vials and connections which are provided by the manufacturer (e.g. vials with transfer connectors) the nurse or whoever is preparing the medication should follow the manufacturer's instructions. The vial now contains a reconstituted solution in which 1 mL = 330 mg.

To calculate the number of millilitres to administer the prescribed dose, you need to convert 265 mg to millilitres:

$$265 \text{ mg} \times \frac{? \text{ mL}}{? \text{ mg}} = ? \text{ mL}$$

The vial contains 330 mg per 1 mL, so the unit fraction is $\dfrac{1 \text{ mL}}{330 \text{ mg}}$:

$$265 \text{ mg} \times \frac{1 \text{ mL}}{330 \text{ mg}} = 0.803 \text{ mL}$$

So, you would withdraw *0.8 mL* (265 mg) from the vial and administer it to the patient.

Practice point

The RCN Standards for Infusion Therapy (2006) sets out a series of good practice standards to minimise errors and dangers, especially in regards to preparing and administering injectable medications. Local policies and risk assessments will indicate what medications can and cannot be reconstituted. Do remember safety and asepsis are paramount.

Practice point

You have a professional responsibility to document all the actions you have taken regarding preparing and administering medications (NMC 2007). After reconstituting a medication, you must label the vial with the date and time of preparation, the amount and type of diluent added, the date and time of expiration of the drug and your name or initials (Smith 2004). When you reconstitute a multidose vial of medication in powdered form, you must also be sure to include the dosage strength on the vial. Once medications are reconstituted, they must be stored and used within the time period indicated in the package insert. Some medications must be reconstituted immediately before administering them because they lose potency rapidly (NPSA 2007). Ampicillin, for example, must be used within 1 hour of being reconstituted.

Stop and think

Suitably qualified nurses ought to routinely flush indwelling infusion devices when not in regular use either with 0.9% sodium chloride or an anticoagulant such as heparin, ensuring that the volume used is at least twice the volume of the catheter. Heparin flush solutions (e.g. Hepsal) are available for maintaining the patency of indwelling intravenous catheters. However, it is recommended that the lowest possible dose of heparin is used to maintain patency, e.g. 10 units in 0.9% sodium chloride (RCN 2006). Do be careful when using heparin: heparin for injection and heparin lock-flush solutions are different drugs and can never be used interchangeably so take care with checking the drug label. Do check your local policy first for safe practice.

Heparin

Heparin sodium is a potent anticoagulant that inhibits clot formation and blood coagulation. Heparin can be administered subcutaneously or intravenously.

Like insulin and some other medications, heparin is supplied and ordered in units. Heparin is available in single and multidose vials, as well as in commercially prepared IV solutions. Heparin is *never given intramuscularly because of the danger of haematomas*. Heparin is available in a variety of strengths, ranging from 10 units/mL to 40 000 units/mL. Heparin is also available in prepackaged syringes. Clexane (enoxaparin) and Fragmin (dalteparin sodium) are examples of low molecular weight heparin. They are used to prevent and treat deep vein thrombosis (DVT) following abdominal surgery, hip or knee replacement, unstable angina or acute coronary syndromes.

Heparin requires close monitoring of the patient's blood count because of the bleeding potential associated with anticoagulant drugs. In order to assure the accuracy of dose measurement, a 1 mL syringe should be used to administer heparin. Nurses and other practitioners administering heparin should be familiar with local policies to ensure safe practice.

Example 8.6

A patient is to have *heparin 2000 units subcutaneously 12 hourly*. The label on the multi-dose vial reads 5000 units/mL. How many millilitres will you administer to the patient? Estimate first – as the available amount is 5000 units per mL it is less than 1 mL. Also, if there are 2500 units in 0.5 mL it will be less than 0.5 mL.

Then continue – you want to convert units to millilitres:

$$2000 \text{ units} = ? \text{ mL}$$

You cancel the units and obtain the equivalent amount in millilitres:

$$2000 \text{ units} \times \frac{? \text{ mL}}{? \text{ units}} = ? \text{ mL}$$

The label on the vial states: '5000 units per millilitre'. So, the unit fraction is

$$\frac{1 \text{ mL}}{5000 \text{ units}}$$

$$2000 \text{ units} \times \frac{1 \text{ mL}}{5000 \text{ units}} = \frac{2 \text{ mL}}{5} = 0.4 \text{ mL}$$

So, you would administer *0.4 mL* of heparin to the patient.

Example 8.7

Another patient is prescribed *heparin 2000 units subcutaneously 12 hourly*. The label on the multidose vial reads 10 000 units/mL. How many millilitres will you administer to the patient?

Again, think logically first to identify the approximate amount. Is it less than 1 mL, less than 0.5 mL? 10 000 units in 1 mL, thus 5000 units in 0.5 mL and 2500 units in 0.25 mL. So you will have an amount less than 0.25 mL.

Continue – you want to convert units to millilitres:

$$2000 \text{ units} = ? \text{ mL}$$

You cancel the units and obtain the equivalent amount in millilitres:

$$2000 \text{ units} \times \frac{? \text{ mL}}{? \text{ units}} = ? \text{ mL}$$

The label on the vial states: '10 000 units per millilitre,' so the unit fraction is $\frac{1 \text{ mL}}{10\,000 \text{ units}}$:

$$2000 \text{ units} \times \frac{1 \text{ mL}}{10\,000 \text{ units}} = \frac{2}{10} = 0.2 \text{ mL}$$

So, you would administer *0.2 mL* of heparin to the patient.

Stop and think

Note that in Examples 8.6 and 8.7 the prescriptions for heparin are exactly the same (2000 units subcutaneously 12 hourly). However, the available dosage strengths are different. In Example 8.7 the strength (10 000 units) is double the strength of that in example 8.6 (5000 units). Therefore, only half the volume of medication is needed. The importance of carefully reading the label must always be considered to determine the correct dose.

Example 8.8

The prescriber orders *dalteparin sodium 120 units/kg subcutaneously 12 hourly* for a patient who weighs 42 kg. See Figure 8.6 and determine how many millilitres of this low molecular weight heparin you will need to administer the dose.

```
          Dalteparin sodium
              Injection
        7,500 IU per 0.3 mL
     For subcutaneous injection
```

Figure 8.6 Drug label for dalteparin sodium

Since this example contains a lot of information, it is useful to summarise it as follows:

Given:	42 kg
Known equivalences:	120 units/kg (prescription)
	7500 units/0.3 mL (strength on the drug label)
Volume you want to find:	? mL

You want to convert a single unit of measurement (42 kg) to another single unit of measurement (mL):

$$42 \text{ kg} = ? \text{ mL}$$

Now, on the left side kg is in the numerator. To cancel the kg will require a unit fraction with kg in the denominator, namely, $\dfrac{120 \text{ units}}{\text{kg}}$:

$$42 \text{ kg} \times \frac{120 \text{ units}}{\text{kg}} = ? \text{ mL}$$

Now, on the left side units is in the numerator. To cancel the units will require a fraction with units in the denominator, namely, $\dfrac{0.3\text{ mL}}{7500\text{ units}}$:

$$42\text{ kg} \times \frac{120\ \cancel{\text{units}}}{\cancel{\text{kg}}} \times \frac{0.3\text{ mL}}{7500\ \cancel{\text{units}}} = ?\text{ mL}$$

Only mL remains on the left side. This is what you want. Now multiply the numbers

$$42\text{ kg} \times \frac{120\ \cancel{\text{units}}}{\cancel{\text{kg}}} \times \frac{0.3\,(\text{mL})}{7500\ \cancel{\text{units}}} = 0.2016\text{ mL}$$

So, if you round up the numbers to one decimal place you will get *0.2 mL.*

Summary

In this chapter, you learned how to calculate doses for administering parenteral medications in liquid form, the procedure for reconstituting medications in powdered form and how to calculate dosages for medications supplied in units.

+ Medications supplied in powdered form must be reconstituted following local policy or the manufacturer's directions.
+ You must determine the best dosage strength for medications ordered when there are several options for reconstituting the medication.
+ Label the medication vial with the date, time and dosage strength after reconstituting a multidose vial.
+ When directions on the label are for IM and IV reconstitution, be sure to read the label carefully to determine the necessary amount of diluent to use.
+ Heparin is measured in units.
+ It is especially important that heparin prescriptions be carefully checked with the heparin type (low molecular weight or regular) and available dosage strength before calculating the amount to be administered.
+ A 1 mL syringe should be used when administering heparin.
+ Heparin sodium and heparin flush solutions are different and should never be used interchangeably.

References

Dougherty, L and Lister, S (eds) *The Royal Marsden Hospital Manual of Clinical Nursing Procedures*, 7th edition. Oxford: Wiley-Blackwell.

Lister S (2008) *Drug Administration General Principles.* In Doughery L and Lister S (eds) *The Royal Marsden Hospital Manual of Clinical Nursing Procedures* 7th edition. Oxford: Blackwell Publishing.

National Patient Safety Agency (NPSA) (2007) *Promoting safer use of injectable medicines Multi-professional safer practice standards for: prescribing, preparing and administering injectable medicines in clinical areas.* London: National Patient Safety Agency. Available at: www.npsa.nhs.uk/health/alerts

Nursing and Midwifery Council (NMC) (2007) *Standards for Medicines Management.* London: Nursing and Midwifery Council.

Royal College of Nursing (RCN) (2006) *Standards for Infusion Therapy.* London: Royal College of Nursing.

Smith J (2004) *Building a Safer NHS for Patients: Improving Medication Safety.* London: HMSO.

Case study 8.1

A 64-year-old man, Mr T, is referred by his general practitioner to the hospital for an emergency appendicectomy following a complaint of abdominal pain, collapse and rapid deterioration. The patient reported a past medical history of hypertension, hypercholesterolaemia and BPH (benign prostatic hypertrophy). He is 1.80 m tall and weighs 68 kg, states he has no known drug or food allergies and is to be imminently transported to the operating theatre. You have completed his admission and his observations indicate: temperature 37.4 °C; B/P 130/86 mmHg; pulse 96/min; resp 18/min. He is huddled over and grimacing, indicating a pain score of 9 (0–10 visual analogue scale) to the lower abdominal area.

In preparation for his impending surgery the patient is assessed for time and type of last meal or food intake (5 hours prior) and liquid intake (sips only more than 2 hours prior); a cannula was sited and intravenous infusion was commenced (Ringers lactate 125 mL/h), morphine 2 mg bolus dose was given for pain.

The plan for post-operative period is as follows:

+ No food orally (nil by mouth or NBM), progress to clear liquids when bowel sounds established and as tolerated
+ Hydration: IV Glucose saline at 125 mL/h
+ Assessment and observations recorded half hourly initially then reduced to 2–4 hourly if stable
+ Antibiotic treatment: metronidazole (Flagyl) 7.5 mg/kg IV infusion 6 hourly and moxifloxacin (Avelox) 400 mg IV daily for 5 days
+ Antihypertensive medication: metoprolol 5 mg IV bolus 4 hourly, omit and report if systolic blood pressure below 110 mmHg or heart rate below 60/min
+ Anticoagulation medication: heparin 5000 units subcutaneously 12 hourly
+ Analgesia for pain: ketorolac (Toradol) 30 mg IM 6 hourly prn for moderate pain
+ Analgesia: oxycodone 5 mg PO 4 hourly prn pain
+ Night sedation: zolpidem (Stilnoct) 5 mg PO before bedtime
+ Hormone antagonist (for BPH): dutasteride (Avodart) 0.5 mg PO every other day

+ Antihypertensive medication: amlodipine (Istin) 10 mg PO daily
+ Antihypertensive medication: enalapril maleate (Innovace) 5 mg PO daily
+ Antihypercholesterolaemia medication: atorvastatin calcium (Lipitor) 20 mg PO every day

Refer to the labels in Figure 8.7 when necessary to answer the following questions.

(a)
```
Metoprolol tartrate
injection for IV use
    5 mg/5 mL
  (5 mL ampoule)
```

(b)
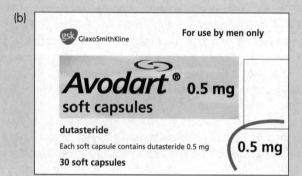

(c)
```
Atorvastin calcium
Tablets 10 mg
```

(d)
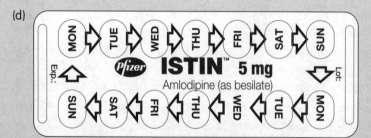

Figure 8.7 Drug labels for Case Study 8.1

[(b) Reproduced with the permission of GlaxoSmithKline; (d) *Reprinted with permission, courtesy of Pfizer Ltd*]

1. The morphine is supplied in ampoules labelled 5 mg/mL.

   (a) How many millilitres are needed for the prescribed dose?

   (b) A 1 mg/mL ampoule costs 72p, a 5 mg/mL ampoule costs £1.30. What would be the cheapest way to provide this injection? Two 1 mg/ml ampoules or one 5 mg/mL ampoule?

2. (a) The heparin vial is labelled 20 000 units/mL. How many millilitres will you prepare?

   (b) Heparin is also available as 5000 units/mL costing: 1 mL ampoule = 54p; 5 mL ampoule = 74p. What is the most cost-effective option in providing this medication?

3. How many millilitres are needed to prepare the IV dose of the metoprolol if the label reads 1 mg/mL?

4. What is the number of milligrams of metronidazole (Flagyl) to be administered?

5. The ketorolac (Toradol) vial is labelled 30 mg/mL. What is the maximum number of millilitres of ketolorac that the patient may receive in 24 hours according to the prescription?

6. Moxifloxacil (Avelox) is supplied in premixed, ready-to-infuse IV bags of 400 mg in 250 mL. How many millilitres will the patient have received in five days?

7. How many capsules of dutasteride will you administer for each dose?

8. How many tablets of amlodipine will you administer each day?

9. The enalopril is supplied in 2.5 mg, 5 mg, 10 mg and 20 mg tablets.

   (a) Which dosage strength will you use?

   (b) How many tablets will you administer?

10. How many tablets of atorvastatin will you administer?

Practice sets

The answers to *Try these for practice*, *Exercises* and *Cumulative review exercises* appear in Appendix A at the end of the book.

Try these for practice

Test your comprehension after reading the chapter.

1. Prescription: *cefuroxime 750 mg IM 8 hourly for 24 hours*. The directions on the 1 g vial of cefuroxime state: 'For IM administration add 2.5 mL of sterile water and shake to provide an approximate volume of 3 mL.'

    (a) How many millilitres will you administer? _____

    (b) What size syringe will you use: 1 mL, 5 mL or 10 mL? _____

2. Prescription: *chlordiazepoxide hydrochloride (Librium) 75 mg IM stat*. The directions on the 100 mg vial state: 'Reconstitute with the 2 mL of special diluent included to provide an approximate volume of 2 mL.'

    (a) How many millilitres will you administer? _____

    (b) What size syringe will you use: 1 mL, 5 mL or 10 mL? _____

3. Prescription: *lorazepam (Ativan) 0.05 mg/kg IM two hours before surgery*. The patient weighs 61 kg, and the label on the 10 mL multidose vial reads: '2 mg per 2 mL.'

    (a) How many milligrams will you prepare? _____

    (b) How many millilitres will you administer (rounded off to two decimal places)? _____

4. Prescription: *heparin 8000 units subcutaneously 12 hourly*. The vial is labelled 10 000 units/mL. How many millilitres will you administer? _____

5. Prescription: *piperacillin sodium 2 g IV stat with probenecid 1 g PO 30 minutes before giving the piperacillin*. The package leaflet for the 2 g piperacillin vial states: 'Add 4 mL of diluent to yield 1 g/2.5 mL.' The label on the probenecid bottle reads: '0.5 g tablet.'

    (a) How many tablets of probenecid will you administer? _____

    (b) How many millilitres of piperacillin contain the prescribed dose? _____

Exercises

Reinforce your understanding in class or at home.

1. The prescriber orders *ampicillin 750 mg IM 6 hourly*. The directions for the 1 g ampicillin vial state 'Reconstitute with 3.5 mL of diluent to yield 250 mg/mL.' How many millilitres will contain the prescribed dose?

2. The prescriber orders *darbepoetin 0.49 mcg/kg subcutaneously once per week* for a patient who weighs 70 kg.

```
Darbepoetin alfa
40 mcg/1 mL
```

Figure 8.8 Drug label for darbepoetin alfa

(a) Read the label in Figure 8.8 and calculate how many millilitres you will administer (rounded off to two decimal places).

(b) What size syringe will you use: 1 mL, 5 mL or 10 mL?_____

3. A patient is prescribed *cefotaxime 1200 mg IM 12 hourly*. The directions on the 1 g vial state: 'Add 3.2 mL of diluent to yield an approximate concentration of 300 mg/mL.' The directions on the 2 g vial state: 'Add 5 mL of diluent to yield an approximate concentration of 330 mg/mL.'

(a) Which vial will you use?

(b) How many millilitres will you administer?

4. The prescriber prescribes *streptomycin 500 mg IM 12 hourly for 7 days*. Read the label in Figure 8.9 and calculate how many millilitres of this antibiotic you will administer.

```
Streptomycin sulphate injection
1 g/2.5 mL
(400 mg/mL)

For IM use ONLY

Store under refrigeration at 2°C–8°C
```

Figure 8.9 Drug label for streptomycin

5. The prescriber orders *etanercept 50 mg subcutaneously once a week.* Read the label in Figure 8.10 and calculate how many vials you will use.

```
Etanercept
25 mg/vial
For subcutaneous use only
```

Figure 8.10 Drug label for etanercept

```
           Epoetin alfa
           20,000 U/mL
         Store at 2°C–8°C
```

Figure 8.11 Drug label for epoetin alfa

6. The prescriber orders *epoetin alfa 6000 units subcutaneously three times a week.* Use the label in Figure 8.11 and do the following:

    (a) Calculate how many millilitres contain the prescribed dose.

    (b) Decide what size syringe you will use to administer this medication: 1 mL, 5 mL or 10 mL?

7. A patient is to have *gentamicin 60 mg IM 12 hourly.* The drug is supplied in a 20 mL multidose vial. The label reads 40 mg/mL. How many millilitres will you administer?

8. The prescriber orders *morphine sulphate 5 mg subcutaneously 4 hourly prn.* The drug is supplied in a 1 mL vial that is labelled 15 mg/mL.

    (a) How many millilitres will you administer?

    (b) What size syringe will you use: 1 mL, 5 mL or 10 mL?

9. A patient needs to have the diuretic *furosemide (Lasix) 30 mg IM stat.* The drug is supplied in a vial labelled 40 mg/mL. How many millilitres will you administer?

10. A patient is to receive *lorazepam (Ativan) 3 mg IM, 2 hours before surgery.* The drug is supplied in a vial labelled 4 mg/mL. How many millilitres will you administer?

11. Use the insulin 'sliding scale' below to determine how much insulin you will give to a patient whose blood glucose is 17 mmol/L (320 mg/dL).

    Order: Give Humulin S unit-100 insulin subcutaneously for blood glucose levels as follows:

    Glucose less than 8 mmol/L (160 mg/dL) – no insulin
    Glucose 8–12 mmol/L (160–220 mmg/dL) – 2 units
    Glucose 12.1–15 mmol/L (221–280 mg/dL) – 4 units
    Glucose 15.1–19 mmol/L (281–340 mg/dL) – 6 units
    Glucose 19.1–22 mmol/L (341–400 mg/dL) – 8 units
    Glucose more than 22 mmol (400 mg/dL) – withhold insulin and call the doctor immediately

12. The prescriber orders *heparin 3500 units subcutaneously 12 hourly.* The label on the vial states 5000 units/mL.

    (a) How many millilitres will you administer?

    (b) What size syringe will you use: 1 mL, 5 mL or 10 mL?

13. A patient is to receive *atropine sulphate 0.2 mg IM 30 minutes before surgery.* The vial is labelled 0.4 mg/mL.

    (a) How many millilitres will you administer?

    (b) What size syringe will you use: 1 mL, 5 mL or 10 mL?

14. Following surgery a patient is prescribed the anti-emetic *promethazine hydrochloride (Phenergan) 12.5 mg IM 4 hourly prn for nausea.* The vial is labelled 50 mg/mL.

    How many millilitres will you administer?

15. The prescriber orders *chlorpromazine hydrochloride 40 mg IM 6 hourly for agitation.* The vial is labelled 25 mg/mL. How many millilitres will you administer?

Cumulative review exercises

Review your mastery of Chapters 5–8.

12. The prescription reads 267 mg/m² of a drug PO. The patient weighs 72 kg and is 178 cm tall. The label reads 50 mg/mL. How many mL will you administer to this patient? Use the nomogram to determine the BSA.

13. A prescriber orders *paracetamol 750 mg PO 8 hourly*. The label reads as follows: Each tablet contains 250 mg. How many tablets will you give this patient?

14. The order reads *Atenolol 100 mg PO daily*. Each tablet contains 0.025 g. How many tablets will you prepare?

15. The physician orders *Bromocriptine mesylate, 7.5 mg PO b.i.d. with meals*. Each tablet contains 2.5 mg. How many tablets of this anti-Parkinsonian drug will you prepare?

16. A patient must receive *60 mmol of potassium chloride PO stat*. Each tablet is labelled 20 mmol/tab. How many tablets will you prepare?

17. Prescription: *add 0.06 g of a drug to 1000 mL of 5% glucose*. Each vial of the drug is labelled 4 mL = 4 mg. How many millilitres of the drug will you add to the 5% glucose?

18. Your patient has an order for a tube feeding of 200 mL of $\frac{3}{4}$ strength Isocal, a nutritional supplement. Each can contains 200 mL of Isocal. How many millilitres of H_2O and how many millilitres of Isocal will you need to make a $\frac{3}{4}$ strength solution? (Hint: $\frac{3}{4}$ strength means 75% solution.)

19. 0.0006 g = _____ mg

20. The prescription reads *atropine sulphate 0.4 mg sc stat*. How many grams will you administer?

21. The prescription is *digoxin 0.25 mg PO q.d.s.* Convert this dose to micrograms.

22. You have 2 mL of Epinephrine (Adrenaline) 1:10 000. How many milligrams of Epinephrine (Adrenaline) are contained in this solution?

Read the label in Figure C.3 to answer questions 23–26.

```
        Quinapril
       hydrochloride
      Tablets 20 mg
     Store below 25°C
```

Figure C.3 Drug label for quinapril

23. What is the generic name of this drug? _____

24. What is the route of administration? _____

25. What are the storage instructions? _____

26. A patient is to receive 80 mg every 12 hours. How many tablets will he receive every 24 hours? _____

27. The prescriber orders betahistine 16 *mg PO daily prn* for vertigo. Read the label in Figure C.4 and calculate how many tablets you will administer.

> Betahistine dihydrochloride
> Tablets 8 mg

Figure C.4 Drug label for betahistine

Read the label in Figure C.5 to answer questions 28–31.

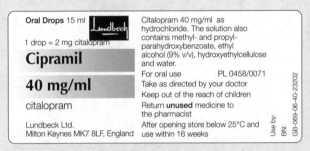

Figure C.5 Drug label for Cipramil
(Courtesy of Lundbeck Ltd)

28. What is the proprietary (trade) name of the drug? _____

29. What is the strength of the drug? _____

30. A patient is to receive 20 mg PO daily. How many millilitres will you administer? _____

31. A patient is to receive 20 mg PO daily. How many doses of medication will this container supply? _____

Unit 3

Infusions and paediatric dosages

Chapter 9

Calculating flow rates and durations of enteral and intravenous infusions

Learning outcomes

After completing this chapter, you will be able to

1. Describe the basic concepts and standard equipment involved in administering enteral and intravenous (IV) infusions.

2. Calculate the flow rates of enteral and IV infusions.

3. Calculate the durations of enteral and IV infusions.

This chapter introduces the basic concepts and standard equipment involved in intravenous and enteral therapy. You will also learn to calculate flow rates for these infusions and to determine how long it will take for a given amount of solution to infuse (its duration).

Diagnostic questions

Before commencing this chapter try to answer the following questions. Compare your answers with those in Appendix A.

1. The rate at which fluids are administered to a patient is in a volume over time (mLs per hour or litres per hour). True or False?

2. Convert 1.5 L of fluid over 6 hours to mLs per hour.

3. Convert 300 mL per hour to mLs per minute.

4. If 1 mL of fluid contains 10 drops, how many drops are there in 50 mL?

5. Flow rate of fluids is in drops per minute. Identify two methods by which this is controlled in clinical settings?

Introduction to intravenous and enteral solutions

Fluids can be given to a patient slowly over a period of time through a vein (**intravenous**) or through a tube inserted into the gastrointestinal tract (**enteral**). The rate at which these fluids flow into the patient is very important and must be controlled precisely.

Enteral feedings

When a patient cannot ingest food or if the upper gastrointestinal tract is not functioning properly, he or she may be prescribed *enteral* feeding ('*tube feeding*'). Enteral feedings provide nutrients and other fluids by way of a tube inserted directly into the gastrointestinal system (alimentary tract).

There are various types of tube feedings. A gastric tube may be inserted into the stomach through the nose (also called nares) (**nasogastric**, as shown in Figure 9.1) or through the mouth (**orogastric**). A longer tube may be similarly inserted, but would extend beyond the stomach into the upper small intestine, jejunum (**nasojejunum** or **orojejunum**).

For long-term feedings, tubes can be inserted surgically or laparoscopically through the wall of the abdomen and directly into either the stomach (**gastrostomy**) or through the stomach and on to the jejunum (**jejunostomy**). These tubes are sutured in place and are referred to as *percutaneous endoscopic gastrostomy (PEG) tubes* and *percutaneous endoscopic jejunostomy (PEJ) tubes*, respectively (see Figure 9.2).

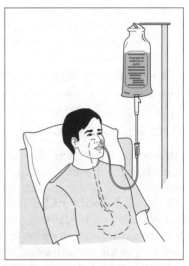

Figure 9.1 A patient with a nasogastric tube

Enteral feedings may be given *continuously* (over a 24-hour period) or *intermittently* (over shorter periods, perhaps several times a day). There are many enteral feeding solutions, including Osmolite, Ensure Plus Fibre, Jevity, Fresubin Resource and Isosource. Enteral feedings are generally administered via pump (see Figure 9.3).

Prescriptions for enteral solutions always indicate a volume of fluid to be infused over a period of time; that is, a flow rate. For example, a tube feeding prescription might read *Jevity 50 mL/h via nasogastric tube for 6 hours beginning 6 A.M.* This prescription is for an

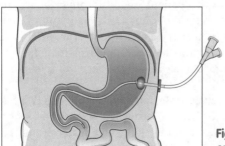

Figure 9.2 A percutaneous endoscopic jejunostomy (PEJ) tube

intermittent feed in which the name of the solution is Jevity, the rate of flow is 50 mL/h, the route of administration is via nasogastric tube and the duration is 6 hours.

> ### Practice point
>
> Make sure you are familiar with your local policy on enteral feeding. You should always check the position of the tube prior to commencing feeding. More information on enteral feeding can be found at: The British Association for Parenteral and Enteral Nutrition.
> (www.bapen.org.uk or www.nutritionsociety.org)

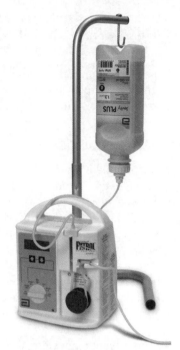

Figure 9.3 Enteral feeding via pump
(Abbott Nutritional Services)

Intravenous infusions

Intravenous (IV) means *through the veins*. Fluids are administered intravenously to provide a variety of fluids, including blood, water containing nutrients, electrolytes, minerals and specific medications to the patient. IV fluids can replace lost fluids, maintain fluid and electrolyte balance or serve as a medium to introduce medications directly into the bloodstream.

Replacement fluids are prescribed for a patient who has lost fluids through haemorrhage, vomiting, or diarrhoea. **Maintenance fluids** help sustain normal levels of fluids and electrolytes. They are prescribed for patients who are at risk of becoming dehydrated or depleted; for example, patients who are to take nothing by mouth (nil by mouth). Furthermore, a patient may be prescribed **parenteral nutrition** which is nutrition fluids administered via an intravenous route, usually a central venous catheter into large veins depending on the duration of therapy (NICE 2006). This is the method used for severely under or malnourished patients (RCN 2005). Parenteral nutrition may provide the full energy requirements (total parenteral nutrition or TPN) or be partial (supplemental parenteral nutrition) where it is not possible to give full requirements or if it may be used in conjunction with enteral feeds. Parenteral nutrition is invasive and has associated risks; therefore it should only be used when there is no alternative method of feeding available and in consultation with the medical team, dietition and pharmacist (BNF 2008). The nutritional fluids vary according to the patient needs (protein, energy or lipds), are administered for continuous or intermittent periods (7–12 hours at a time) and are generally prepared aseptically by the pharmacy department. The RCN (2005) have included parenteral feeding under the guidance called: Standards for Infusion Therapy (standard 8.5). The principles of calculations apply equally to parenteral feeding as other infusion therapies.

Intravenous infusions may be **continuous** or **intermittent**. Continuous IV infusions are used to replace or maintain fluids or electrolytes. Intermittent IV infusions – for example, IV accessory infusion tubes or Y or 3-way ports – are used to administer drugs and supplemental fluids. *Intermittent peripheral infusion devices* (saline locks or heparin locks) are used to maintain venous access without continuous fluid infusion. Intermittent IV infusions are discussed in Chapter 10.

A healthcare professional must be able to perform the calculations to determine the correct rate at which an enteral or intravenous solution will enter the body (**flow rate**). Infusion flow rates are usually measured in drops per minute (drops/min) or millilitres per hour (mL/h). It is important to be able to convert each of these rates to the other and to determine how long a given amount of solution will take to infuse.

For example, an IV prescription might read *IV fluids: glucose 5% over 8 hours*. In this case, the prescription is for an IV infusion in which the name of the solution is 5% glucose, the route of administration is intravenous and the duration is 8 hours. Alternatively, the prescription might read *IV fluids: glucose 5% 125 mL/h*. In this case, the prescription is for an IV infusion, the flow rate is 125 mL/h and the route of administration is intravenous. There are other ways to assist in understanding the calculations for this:

$$\text{hourly flow rate} = \frac{\text{total amount of IV fluid}}{\text{number of hours for infusion}}$$

e.g. 1 L of normal saline is prescribed to be infused over 8 hours:

$$\text{hourly rate} = \frac{1000 \text{ mL}}{8 \text{ h}} = 125 \text{ mL}$$

Practice point

Aspetic technique is important with all types of fluid infusions, both the infusion or cannula site and the closed system for IV fluid administration. Some fluids can be given for long periods of time (continuous) and others for short periods of time (intermittent). It is important to monitor the fluids given to patients, especially if IV or via nasogastric tubes, and report if the patient is having fluid too fast or too much as this may lead to problems (e.g overload).

Intravenous solutions

A **saline solution**, which is a solution of *sodium chloride (NaCl)* in sterile water, is commonly used for intravenous infusion. Sodium chloride is ordinary table salt. Saline solutions are available in various concentrations for different purposes. A 0.9% NaCl solution is referred to as **normal saline (NS)**. Intravenous fluids generally contain glucose, sodium chloride and/or electrolytes:

+ 5% glucose solution, which means that 5 g of glucose are dissolved in water to make each 100 mL of this solution (see Figures 9.4a and 9.4b).
+ 0.9% NaCl is a solution in which each 100 mL contain 0.9 g of sodium chloride (see Figures 9.4c and 9.4d).
+ Replacement of normal body fluids (Figures 9.5b and 9.5d): 5% glucose and 0.45% sodium chloride, 4% glucose and 0.18% sodium chloride.
+ Some with electrolytes (Figures 9.5a and 9.5c): potassium 0.15% with glucose 4%, 5% glucose and Ringers lactate.

Additional information on IV fluids can be found in nursing and pharmacology textbooks.

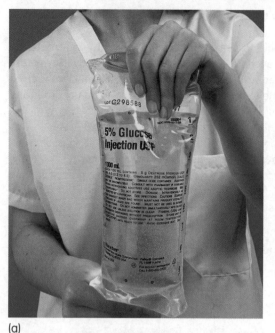

(a)

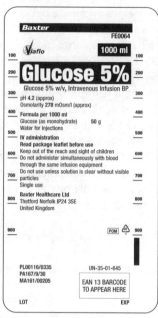

(b)

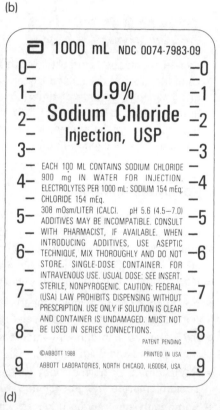

(c)

(d)

Figure 9.4 Examples of IV bags and labels

((a) Al Dodge/Al Dodge (b) Courtesy of Baxter Healthcare Ltd. All rights reserved (c) Al Dodge/Al Dodge Photography (d) Reproduced with permission of Abbott Laboratories)

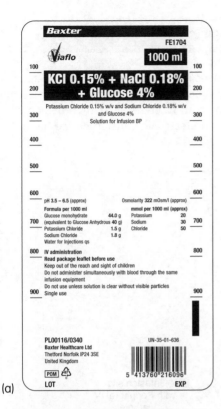

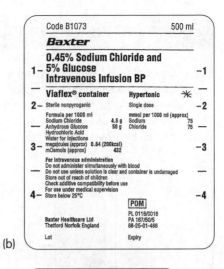

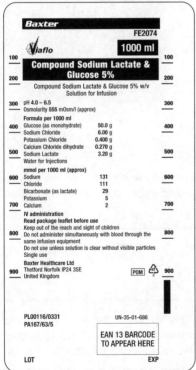

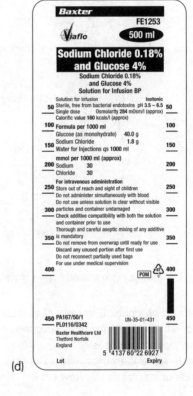

Figure 9.5 Examples of intravenous fluids

Equipment for intravenous infusions

Equipment used for the administration of continuous IV infusions includes the IV solution and IV tubing ('giving set'), a drip chamber, at least one injection port and a roller clamp. The tubing connects the IV solution to the hub of an IV catheter at the infusion site. The rate of flow of the infusion is regulated by an electronic infusion device (pump or controller) or by gravity (see Figures 9.6 and 9.9).

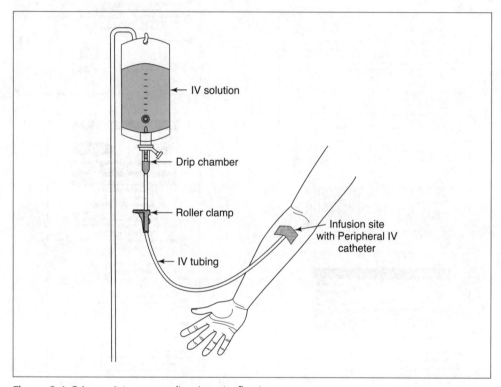

Figure 9.6 Primary intravenous line (gravity flow)

The drip chamber (Figure 9.6) is located at the site of the entrance of the tubing into the container of intravenous solution. It allows you to count the number of drops per minute that the client is receiving (flow rate).

A roll valve clamp or clip is connected to the tubing and can be manipulated to increase or decrease the flow rate.

Practice point

Be sure to follow the procedures for eliminating all air in the tubing. Maintain aseptic procedures at all stages of the preparations. This equipment is invasive and it could be potentially harmful to a patient if infection or air enters into a vein.

The size of the drop that IV tubing delivers is not standard; it depends on the way the tubing is designed (see Figure 9.7). Manufacturers specify the number of drops that are equal to 1 mL for their particular tubing. This is called the tubing's **drop factor** (see Figure 9.8 and Table 9.1). You must know the tubing's drop factor when calculating the flow rate of solutions in drops per minute (dpm) or microdrops per minute (μdpm or mcdpm). If in doubt always look at the packaging of the IV giving set. This does add another aspect to the calculation which will require practice.

Figure 9.7 Tubing with drip chamber
(Photodisc/Getty Images)

Infusion pumps

An intravenous infusion can flow solely by the force of gravity or by an electronic infusion device. There are many different types of electronic infusion machines, including controllers and volumetric pumps (see Figure 9.9).

These electrically operated devices allow the rate of flow (usually specified in mL/h) to be simply keyed into the device by the user. The pumps can regulate the flow rate more precisely than the gravity systems can. For example, pumps detect an interruption in the flow (constriction) and sound an alarm to alert the nursing staff and the patient, sound an alarm when the infusion finishes, indicate the volume of fluid already infused and indicate the time remaining for the infusion to finish. 'Smart' pumps may contain libraries of safe dosage ranges that will not allow the user to key in an unsafe dosage.

A **patient controlled analgesia (PCA)** pump (see Figure 9.10) allows a patient to self-administer pain-relieving drugs whenever the patient needs them without having to wait for the nurse to bring medication. When pain is felt, the patient presses the button on the handset, which is connected to the PCA pump. The pump then delivers the drug down a length of tubing to an injection port.

Table 9.1 Common drop factors

10 drops = 1 mL ⎫
15 drops = 1 mL ⎬ macrodrops
20 drops = 1 mL ⎭
60 micro drops = 60 μdrops = 1 mL } microdrops

Practice point

A clinical area might use many different types of infusion pumps. The nurse or practitioner must learn how to set up and use all of them. Be sure to use the specific tubing supplied by the manufacturer for each pump. There could be a danger in the patient receiving an incorrect amount of drug: too much or too little, either of which may be harmful, e.g too much heparin and a consequent risk of bleeding.

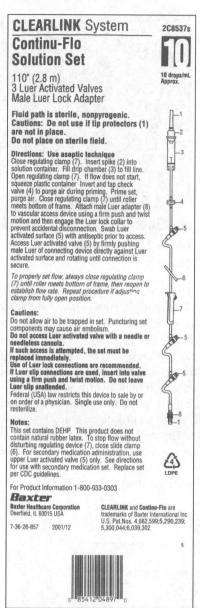

CLEARLINK System   2C8537s

Continu-Flo
Solution Set

10
10 drops/mL
Approx.

110" (2.8 m)
3 Luer Activated Valves
Male Luer Lock Adapter

**Fluid path is sterile, nonpyrogenic.
Cautions: Do not use if tip protectors (1)
are not in place.
Do not place on sterile field.**

Directions: Use aseptic technique
Close regulating clamp (7). Insert spike (2) into
solution container. Fill drip chamber (3) to fill line.
Open regulating clamp (7). If flow does not start,
squeeze plastic container Invert and tap check
valve (4) to purge air during priming. Prime set,
purge air. Close regulating clamp (7) until roller
meets bottom of frame. Attach male Luer adapter (8)
to vascular access device using a firm push and twist
motion and then engage the Luer lock collar to
prevent accidental disconnection. Swab Luer
activated surface (5) with antiseptic prior to access.
Access Luer activated valve (5) by firmly pushing
male Luer of connecting device directly against Luer
activated surface and rotating until connection is
secure.

*To properly set flow, always close regulating clamp
(7) until roller meets bottom of frame, then reopen to
establish flow rate. Repeat procedure if adjusting
clamp from fully open position.*

Cautions:
Do not allow air to be trapped in set. Puncturing set
components may cause air embolism.
**Do not access Luer activated valve with a needle or
needleless cannula.
If such access is attempted, the set must be
replaced immediately.
Use of Luer lock connections are recommended.
If Luer slip connections are used, insert into valve
using a firm push and twist motion. Do not leave
Luer slip unattended.**
Federal (USA) law restricts this device to sale by or
on order of a physician. Single use only. Do not
resterilize.

Notes:
This set contains DEHP. This product does not
contain natural rubber latex. To stop flow without
disturbing regulating device (7), close slide clamp
(6). For secondary medication administration, use
upper Luer activated valve (5) only. See directions
for use with secondary medication set. Replace set
per CDC guidelines.

For Product Information 1-800-933-0303

Baxter

Baxter Healthcare Corporation
Deerfield, IL 60015 USA

7-36-26-857   2001/12

CLEARLINK and **Continu-Flo** are
trademarks of Baxter International Inc.
U.S. Pat.Nos. 4,662,599;5,290,239;
5,300,044;6,039,302

5

0 85412 04897 0

(a)

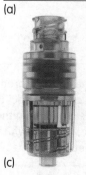

(c)

2C7524 s

Baxter

Buretrol®
Solution Set

150 mL Burette
Burette Chamber Filter Valve
Injection Site
Flashball® Device

60

60 drops approx. 1 mL

2.1 m (84") long

*Sterile, nonpyrogenic fluid path

**Caution: Federal (USA) law restricts this device
to sale by or on order of a physician.**

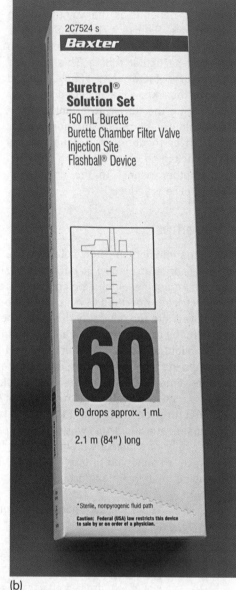

(b)

Figure 9.8 Samples of IV tubing containers
with drop factors of 10 and 60

((a) Images provided courtesy of Baxter Healthcare Corporation.
All rights reserved (b) Al Dodge/Al Dodge Photography
(c) Courtesy of Baxter Healthcare Ltd)

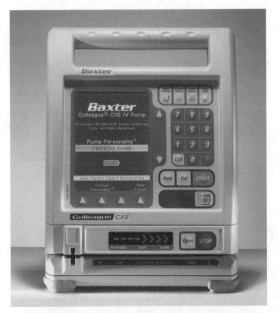

Figure 9.9 Volumetric infusion pump
(Courtesy of Baxter Healthcare Ltd)

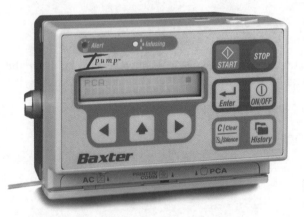

Figure 9.10 PCA pump
(Courtesy of Baxter Healthcare Ltd)

Calculating the flow rate of infusions

In the following examples, you will be required to change one rate of flow to another rate of flow. The general method for converting one rate to another rate was introduced in Chapter 3. To recap:

+ Start with the unit of measure you have on the left side of the = sign.
+ Write the unit of measure you want to *find* on the right side of the = sign.
+ Identify an *equivalence* containing the units of measure in the problem.
+ Use the equivalence to make a unit fraction with the unit you have as the *denominator*.
+ Multiply by the unit fraction.

197

+ Cancel the units of measure. The only unit of measurement remaining on the left side (in a numerator) will match the unit of measure on the right side.
+ Cancel the numbers and finish the multiplication.

Example 9.1

The order is *glucose saline 1250 mL IV 12 hourly*. The tubing is calibrated at 10 drops per millilitre. Calculate the number of drops per minute that you would administer.

Given flow rate:	1250 mL/12 h
Known equivalences:	10 drops/mL (drop factor)
	1 h = 60 min
Flow rate you want to find:	? drops/min

You want to convert one flow rate in mL/h to an equivalent flow rate in drops/min:

$$\frac{1250 \text{ mL}}{12 \text{ h}} = \frac{? \text{ drops}}{\text{min}}$$

You want to cancel mL. To do this you must use a unit fraction containing mL in the denominator. Using the drop factor, this fraction will be $\frac{10 \text{ drops}}{1 \text{ mL}}$:

$$\frac{1250 \text{ mL}}{12 \text{ h}} \times \frac{10 \text{ drops}}{1 \text{ mL}} = \frac{? \text{ drops}}{\text{min}}$$

Now, on the left side *drops* is in the numerator, which is what you want. But *h* is in the denominator and it must be cancelled. This will require a unit fraction with *h* in the numerator, namely, $\frac{1 \text{ h}}{60 \text{ min}}$. Now, cancel and multiply the numbers:

$$\frac{1250 \text{ mL}}{12 \text{ h}} \times \frac{10 \text{ drops}}{1 \text{ mL}} \times \frac{1 \text{ h}}{60 \text{ min}} = 17.4 \frac{\text{drops}}{\text{min}}$$

So, the flow rate is *17 drops per minute*.

Example 9.2

The prescription states *IV fluids: 0.9% NaCl 250 mL in 4 hours*. The giving set you are using has a drop rate of 60 drops/mL (microdrops). How many microdrops per minute would you administer?

Given flow rate:	250 mL/4 h
Known equivalences:	60 mcdrops/mL (drop factor)
	1 h = 60 min
Flow rate you want to find:	? mcdrops/min

You want to convert one flow rate in mL/h to an equivalent flow rate in mcdrops/min:

$$\frac{250 \text{ mL}}{4 \text{ h}} = \frac{? \text{ mcdrops}}{\text{min}}$$

You want to cancel mL. To do this you must use a unit fraction containing mL in the denominator. Using the drop factor, this fraction will be $\dfrac{60\ \text{mcdrop}}{1\ \text{mL}}$:

$$\frac{250\ \text{mL}}{4\ \text{h}} \times \frac{60\ \text{drops}}{1\ \text{mL}} = \frac{?\ \text{mcdrops}}{\text{min}}$$

Now, on the left side *mcdrop* is in the numerator, which is what you want. But *h* is in the denominator and it must be cancelled. This will require a fraction with *h* in the numerator, namely, $\dfrac{1\ \text{h}}{60\ \text{min}}$. Now, cancel and multiply the numbers:

$$\frac{250\ \text{mL}}{4\ \text{h}} \times \frac{60\ \text{drops}}{1\ \text{mL}} \times \frac{1\ \text{h}}{60\ \text{min}} = 62.5\ \frac{\text{drops}}{\text{min}}$$

So, *63 microdrops per minute* would be administered.

> **Note**
>
> Continuous enteral feedings are generally placed on an infusion pump and measured in mL/h.

> **Stop and think**
>
> When starting these calculations put what you *have* on the left of the equals sign and the units you *wish to find* (e.g. mL/h or drops/min) on the right. Use a stepwise process to cancel and multiply the elements you put in place. Always double check your answers to ensure patient safety (avoid over or under loading of fluids).

Example 9.3

A patient must receive a nasogastric tube-feeding of *Ensure, 240 mL in 90 minutes*. The calibration of the tubing is 20 drops per millilitre. Calculate the flow rate in millilitres per hour.

Given flow rate:	240 mL/90 min
Known equivalences:	20 drops/mL (drop factor)
	1 h = 60 min
Flow rate you want to find:	? mL/h

You want to change one flow rate to another:

$$\frac{240\ \text{mL}}{90\ \text{min}} = \frac{?\ \text{mL}}{\text{h}}$$

Each side has *mL* in the numerator, which is what you want. You want to cancel *min* which is in the denominator. To do this you must use a unit fraction containing *min* in the numerator. This fraction will be $\dfrac{60 \text{ min}}{1 \text{ h}}$:

$$\frac{240\,\cancel{\text{mL}}}{9\cancel{0}\,\cancel{\text{min}}} \times \frac{6\cancel{0}\,\cancel{\text{min}}}{1\,\text{h}} = 160\,\frac{\text{mL}}{\text{h}}$$

So, the flow rate is *160 mL per hour.*

Example 9.4

A client is prescribed *normal saline (0.9% NaCl) 850 mL IV in 8 hours.* The label on the box containing the intravenous giving set to be used for this infusion is shown in Figure 9.11. Calculate the flow rate in drops per minute.

Given flow rate: 850 mL/8 h

Known equivalences: 10 drops/mL (drop factor)

 1 h = 60 min

Flow rate you want to find: ? drops/min

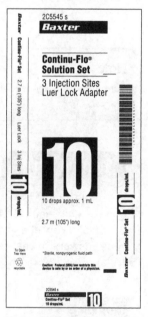

Figure 9.11 Continu-Flo Solution Set box label

(Images provided courtesy of Baxter Healthcare Corporation)

You want to convert the flow rate from millilitres per hour to drops per minute:

$$\frac{850 \text{ mL}}{8 \text{ h}} = \frac{? \text{ drops}}{\text{min}}$$

You want to cancel mL. To do this you must use a unit fraction containing mL in the denominator. Using the drop factor, this fraction will be $\dfrac{10 \text{ drops}}{1 \text{ mL}}$:

$$\frac{850\,\cancel{\text{mL}}}{8 \text{ h}} \times \frac{10 \text{ drops}}{1\,\cancel{\text{mL}}} = \frac{? \text{ drops}}{\text{min}}$$

Now, on the left side *drops* is in the numerator, which is what you want. But *h* is in the denominator and it must be cancelled. This will require a unit fraction with *h* in the numerator, namely, $\dfrac{1 \text{ h}}{60 \text{ min}}$. Now cancel and multiply the numbers:

$$\frac{850\,\cancel{\text{mL}}}{8\,\cancel{\text{h}}} \times \frac{10\,\cancel{\text{drops}}}{1\,\cancel{\text{mL}}} \times \frac{1\,\cancel{\text{h}}}{6\cancel{0}\,\cancel{\text{min}}} = 17.7\,\frac{\text{drops}}{\text{min}}$$

So, the flow rate is *18 drops per minute.*

Stop and think

Sometimes, for a variety of reasons, the infusion flow rate can change. A change may affect the prescribed duration of time in which the solution will be administered. For example, with a gravity system, raising or lowering the infusion site or moving the patient's body or bed relative to the height of the bag may change the flow rate of the IV infusion. Therefore, the flow rate must be assessed regularly, and adjustments made if necessary. Examples 9.5 and 9.6 illustrate the computations involved in this process.

Example 9.5

1. The order is *500 mL of 5% glucose to infuse IV in 5 hours*. Calculate the flow rate in drops per minute if the drop factor is 15 drops per millilitre.

2. When the nurse checks the infusion 2 hours after it started, 400 mL remain to be infused in the remaining 3 hours. Recalculate the flow rate in drops per minute for the remaining 400 mL.

1. Given flow rate: 500 mL/5 h

   Known equivalences: 15 drops/mL (drop factor)

                                  1 h = 60 min

   Flow rate you want to find: ? drops/min

You want to convert the flow rate from 500 mL in 5 hours to drops per minute:

$$\frac{500 \text{ mL}}{5 \text{ h}} = ? \frac{\text{drops}}{\text{min}}$$

As in the previous examples, you can do this in one line as follows:

$$\frac{500 \text{ mL}}{5 \text{ h}} \times \frac{15 \text{ drops}}{1 \text{ mL}} \times \frac{1 \text{ h}}{60 \text{ min}} = 25 \frac{\text{drops}}{\text{min}}$$

So, the flow rate is *25 drops per minute*.

2. When the nurse checks the infusion, 400 mL need to be infused in 3 hours.

   So, you now want to convert 400 mL in 3 hours to drops per minute:

$$\frac{400 \text{ mL}}{3 \text{ h}} = \frac{? \text{ drops}}{\text{min}}$$

In a similar manner to part (a), you can do this in one line as follows:

$$\frac{400 \text{ mL}}{3 \text{ h}} \times \frac{15 \text{ drops}}{1 \text{ mL}} \times \frac{1 \text{ h}}{60 \text{ min}} = 33.3 \frac{\text{drops}}{\text{min}}$$

So, in order for the infusion to be completed within the 5 hour time period as prescribed, the flow rate must be increased to *33 drops per minute*.

Example 9.6

The prescription is *glucose 900 mL IV in 6 hours*. The drop factor is 10 drop/mL. You would expect that after 3 hours, about 450 mL (half the total infusion of 900 mL) would be left in the bag. However, only 240 mL remain. Recalculate the flow rate in drops/min so that the infusion will finish on time.

The remainder of the bag (240 mL) must infuse in the remaining time (3 hours).

New flow rate:	240 mL/3 h
Known equivalences:	10 drops/mL (drop factor)
	1 h = 60 min
Flow rate you want to find:	? drops/min

You want to convert the flow rate from 240 mL in 3 hours to drops per minute:

$$\frac{240 \text{ mL}}{3 \text{ h}} = \frac{? \text{ drops}}{\text{min}}$$

You can do this in one line as follows:

$$\frac{240 \text{ mL}}{3 \text{ h}} \times \frac{10 \text{ drops}}{1 \text{ mL}} \times \frac{1 \text{ h}}{60 \text{ min}} = 13.3 \frac{\text{drops}}{\text{min}}$$

So, the new flow rate would be *13 drops per minute*.

Always double check your answers to safeguard the patients from harmful drug or fluid flow rates (too fast or too slow). One way to double check is using the following:

$$\frac{\text{drops}}{\text{min}} = \frac{\text{drops/mL of giving set} \times \text{volume of the infusion}}{\text{Number of mins the infusion is to run}}$$

Using the previous example:

$$\frac{10 \text{ drops/mL} \times 240 \text{ mL}}{180 \text{ min}} = 13.3 \text{ drops/min}$$

Example 9.7

A patient has an order for *Fresubin 240 mL over 2 hours via a feeding tube*. Calculate the rate of flow in:

1. millilitres per hour

2. millilitres per minute.

1. The flow rate is 240 mL in 2 hours. No conversion of units of measurement is necessary. $\frac{240 \text{ mL}}{2 \text{ h}}$ can be simplified as follows:

$$\frac{\overset{120}{\cancel{240}} \text{ mL}}{\underset{1}{\cancel{2} \text{ h}}} = \frac{120 \text{ mL}}{\text{h}}$$

So, the flow rate is *120 mL* per hour.

2. Change the flow rate found in part (a) to millilitres per minute. You want to convert the millilitres per hour into millilitres per minute:

$$\frac{120 \text{ mL}}{\text{h}} = \frac{? \text{ mL}}{\text{min}}$$

Do this in one line as follows:

$$\frac{120 \text{ mL}}{\cancel{h}} \times \frac{1 \cancel{h}}{60 \text{ min}} = 2 \frac{\text{mL}}{\text{min}}$$

So, the flow rate is *2 mL per minute*.

Example 9.8

The prescriber orders 4% *glucose/0.18% NaCl IV* to infuse at *21 drops per minute*. If the drop factor is 20 drops per millilitre, how many millilitres per hour will the patient receive?

Given flow rate:	21 drops/min
Known equivalences:	20 drops/mL (drop factor)
	1 h = 60 min
Flow rate you want to find:	? mL/h

You want to convert a flow rate of 21 drops per minute to a flow rate in millilitres per hour:

$$\frac{21 \text{ drops}}{\text{min}} = \frac{? \text{ mL}}{\text{h}}$$

You want to cancel drops. To do this you must use a unit fraction containing drops in the denominator. Using the drop factor, this fraction is $\frac{1 \text{ mL}}{20 \text{ drops}}$:

$$\frac{21 \text{ drops}}{\text{min}} \times \frac{1 \text{ mL}}{20 \text{ drops}} = \frac{? \text{ mL}}{\text{h}}$$

Now, on the left side mL is in the numerator, which is what you want. But min is in the denominator and it must be cancelled. This will require a unit fraction with min in the numerator, namely, $\frac{60 \text{ min}}{1 \text{ h}}$. Now cancel and multiply the numbers:

$$\frac{21 \cancel{\text{drops}}}{\cancel{\text{min}}} \times \frac{1 \cancel{\text{mL}}}{20 \cancel{\text{drops}}} \times \frac{60 \cancel{\text{min}}}{1 \cancel{\text{h}}} = 63 \frac{\text{mL}}{\text{h}}$$

So, the flow rate is *63 mL per hour*.

Stop and think

As an example, 125 mL per hour is the same flow rate as 125 microdrops per minute because the 60s always cancel. The flow rates of *millilitres per hour* and *microdrops per minute* are equivalent. Therefore calculations are not always necessary to change mL/h to mcdrops/min. It is important to note this is only if the giving set used is calibrated at 60 drops/mL

Calculating the duration of flow for intravenous and enteral solutions

In the following four examples, you must determine the length of time it will take to complete an infusion.

Example 9.9

An infusion of 5% glucose is infusing at a rate of 20 drops per minute. If the drop factor is 12 drops per millilitre, how many hours will it take for the remaining solution in the bag (Figure 9.12) to infuse?

In Figure 9.12 you can see that 500 mL of solution were originally in the bag, and that the patient has received 200 mL. Therefore, 300 mL remain to be infused.

Given: 300 mL (volume to be infused)

Known

equivalences: 12 drops/mL (drop factor)

20 drops/min (flow rate)

1 h = 60 min

Find: ? h

You want to convert this single unit of measurement 300 mL to the single unit of measurement *hours*:

$$300 \text{ mL} = ? \text{ h}$$

You want to cancel mL. To do this you must use a unit fraction containing mL in the denominator. Using the drop factor, this fraction will be $\dfrac{12 \text{ drops}}{1 \text{ mL}}$:

$$300 \text{ mL} \times \frac{12 \text{ drops}}{1 \text{ mL}} = ? \text{ h}$$

Figure 9.12
5% Glucose intravenous solution

Now, on the left side drops is in the numerator, but you don't want drops. You need a unit fraction with drops in the denominator to cancel. Using the flow rate, this fraction is $\dfrac{1 \text{ min}}{20 \text{ drops}}$:

$$300 \; \cancel{mL} \times \frac{12 \; \cancel{drops}}{1 \; \cancel{mL}} \times \frac{1 \; \textcircled{min}}{20 \; \cancel{drops}} = ? \, h$$

Now, on the left side min is in the numerator, but you don't want min. You need a fraction with min in the denominator to cancel, namely, $\dfrac{1 \text{ h}}{60 \text{ min}}$. Now cancel and multiply the numbers:

$$\overset{15}{\cancel{300}} \; \cancel{mL} \times \frac{\overset{1}{\cancel{12}} \; \cancel{drops}}{1 \; \cancel{mL}} \times \frac{1 \; \cancel{min}}{\underset{1}{\cancel{20}} \; \cancel{drops}} \times \frac{1 \; h}{\underset{5}{\cancel{60}} \; \cancel{min}} = 3 \, h$$

So, it will take *3 hours* for the remaining solution to infuse.

(**Example 9.10**)

A patient is to receive an IV infusion of 500 mL of 5% glucose. The flow rate is 27 drops per minute. If the drop factor is 15 drops per millilitre, how many hours will it take for this infusion to finish?

Given:	500 mL (volume to be infused)
Known equivalences:	15 drops/mL (drop factor)
	27 drops/min (flow rate)
	1 h = 60 min
Find:	? h

You want to convert this single unit of measurement 500 mL to the single unit of measurement *hours*:

$$500 \text{ mL} = ? \, h$$

You want to cancel mL. To do this you must use a unit fraction containing mL in the denominator. Using the drop factor, this fraction will be $\dfrac{15 \text{ drops}}{1 \text{ mL}}$:

$$500 \text{ mL} \times \frac{15 \text{ drops}}{1 \text{ mL}} = ? \, h$$

Now, on the left side drops is in the numerator, but you don't want drops. You need a unit fraction with drops in the denominator. Using the flow rate, the fraction is $\dfrac{1 \text{ min}}{27 \text{ drops}}$:

$$500 \; \cancel{mL} \times \frac{15 \; \cancel{drops}}{1 \; \cancel{mL}} \times \frac{1 \; \textcircled{min}}{27 \; \cancel{drops}} = ? \, h$$

Now, on the left side min is in the numerator, but you don't want min. You need a unit fraction with min in the denominator, namely, $\dfrac{1\ h}{60\ min}$. Now cancel and multiply the numbers:

$$500\ \cancel{mL} \times \frac{\overset{1}{\cancel{15}}\ \cancel{drops}}{1\ \cancel{mL}} \times \frac{1\ \cancel{min}}{27\ \cancel{drops}} \times \frac{1\ h}{\underset{4}{\cancel{60}}\ \cancel{min}} = 4.63\ h$$

Now, convert the portion of an hour to minutes – that is, convert 0.63 h to min. Use a fraction with h as a denominator so you can cancel this out then multiply the numbers:

$$0.63\ \cancel{h} \times \frac{60\ min}{1\ \cancel{h}} = 37.8\ min$$

So, the infusion will take *4 hours and 38 minutes*.

(**Example 9.11**)

An IV of 1000 mL of 0.9% NaCl is started at 20.00 h (8 P.M). The flow rate is 38 drops per minute and the drop factor is 10 drops per millilitre. At what time will this infusion finish?

Given: 1000 mL (volume to be infused)

Known equivalences: 10 drops/mL (drop factor)

                                       38 drops/min (flow rate)

                                       1 h = 60 min

Find: ? h

You must first find how many hours the infusion will take to finish. You want to convert the single unit of measurement 1000 mL to the single unit of measurement *hours*:

$$1000\ mL = ?\ h$$

You want to cancel mL. To do this you must use a unit fraction containing mL in the denominator. This fraction will be $\dfrac{10\ drops}{1\ mL}$:

$$1000\ \cancel{mL} \times \frac{10\ drops}{1\ \cancel{mL}} = ?\ h$$

Now, on the left side drops is in the numerator, but you don't want drops. You need a fraction with drops in the denominator. Using the flow rate, this fraction is $\dfrac{1\ min}{38\ drops}$:

$$1000\ \cancel{mL} \times \frac{10\ \cancel{drops}}{1\ \cancel{mL}} \times \frac{1\ \boxed{min}}{38\ \cancel{drops}} = ?\ h$$

Now, on the left side min is in the numerator, but you don't want min. You need a fraction with min in the denominator, namely, $\dfrac{1\ h}{60\ min}$. Now, cancel and multiply the numbers:

$$1000 \ \cancel{mL} \times \frac{\overset{1}{\cancel{10 \ drops}}}{1 \ \cancel{mL}} \times \frac{1 \ \cancel{min}}{38 \ \cancel{drops}} \times \frac{1 \ h}{\underset{6}{\cancel{60 \ min}}} = 4.4 \ h$$

You then convert 0.4 h to min:

$$0.4 \ \cancel{h} \times \frac{60 \ min}{1 \ \cancel{h}} = 24 \ min$$

So, the IV will infuse for 4 hours and 24 minutes. Because the infusion started at 8 P.M., it will finish at *00.24 (12:24 A.M.) on the following day.*

Example 9.12

The prescription reads *1000 mL glucose 5% IV over 8 hours.* The drop factor is 10 drops/mL.

1. Calculate the flow rate in drops/min for this infusion.
2. After 5 hours 700 mL remain to be infused. How must the flow rate be adjusted so that the infusion will finish on time?
3. If the clinical area has a policy that flow rate adjustments must not exceed 25% of the original rate, was the adjustment required within the policy guidelines?

1. First, convert the flow rate of 1000 mL in 8 hours to drops/min. You can do this in one line as follows:

$$\frac{1000 \ \cancel{mL}}{8 \ \cancel{h}} \times \frac{1 \ \cancel{h}}{60 \ min} \times \frac{10 \ drops}{\cancel{mL}} = 20.8 \ \frac{drops}{min}$$

So, the original flow rate is *21 drops/min.*

2. After 5 hours, 700 mL remain to be infused in the remaining 3 hours. Now, the new flow rate must be calculated. That is, you must convert the flow rate of 700 mL in 3 hours to drops/min. You can do this in one line as follows:

$$\frac{700 \ \cancel{mL}}{3 \ \cancel{h}} \times \frac{1 \ \cancel{h}}{60 \ min} \times \frac{10 \ drops}{\cancel{mL}} = 38.9 \ \frac{drops}{min}$$

So, the new flow rate is *39 drops/min.*

3. Since the facility has a policy that flow rate adjustments must not exceed 25% of the original rate, you must now calculate 25% of the original rate; that is, 25% of 21 drops/min:

$$25\% \ of \ 21 \ drops/min = (0.25 \times 21) \ drops/min = 5.25 \ drops/min$$

So, the flow rate may not be changed by more than about 5 drops/min. Therefore, the original flow rate of 21 drops/min can be changed to no less than 16 (21 minus 5) drops/min and no more than 26 (21 plus 5) drops/min.

Since 39 drops/min is outside the acceptable range of roughly 16–26 drops/min, this change is not within the guidelines, and the adjustment may not be made. You must contact the nurse in charge and the prescriber.

Practice point

Whilst it is important to get the calculations correct, it is also important to ensure you have the correct information (infusions, equipment, prescription instructions, etc.). According to the RCN Guidelines for Infusion Therapy (2005) Standard 9.9, prescribed intravenous fluids should be administered over the specified time in order to prevent speed shock and fluid overload which is a dangerous complication of incorrect fluid administration (too fast) (Lister 2008). The nurse ought to make regular observations of IV fluids to ensure potentially dangerous 'speeding up' of fluids does not happen.

Summary

In this chapter, the basic concepts and standard equipment involved in intravenous and enteral therapy were introduced.

+ Fluids can be given to a patient slowly over a period of time through a vein (*intravenous*) or through a tube inserted into the gastrointestinal tract (*enteral*).
+ Enteral and IV fluids can be administered continuously or intermittently.
+ There is a wide variety of commercially prepared enteral and IV solutions.
+ Care must be taken to eliminate the air from, and maintain the sterility of, IV giving set tubing.
+ An intravenous infusion can flow solely by the force of gravity or by an electronic infusion device.
+ Flow rates are usually given as either mL/h or drops/min.
+ To find the flow rate in *mL/h*, start with the flow rate in *drops/min*.
+ To find the flow rate in *drops/min*, start with the flow rate in *mL/h*.
+ The drop factor of the IV administration giving set must be known in order to calculate flow rates.
+ *Microdrops/minute* are equivalent to *millilitres/hour*.
+ For microdrops, the drop factor is 60 microdrops per millilitre.
+ For macrodrops, the usual drop factors are 10, 15 or 20 drops per millilitre.
+ To calculate the duration of an IV infusion, start with the volume of the solution in the bag.
+ Know the local policy regarding readjustment of flow rates.
+ Useful formulae to remember (once you have mastered the calculation process):

$$\text{hourly flow rate} = \frac{\text{total amount of IV fluid}}{\text{number of hours for infusion}}$$

$$\text{drops/min} = \frac{\text{drops/mL of giving set} \times \text{volume of the infusion}}{\text{number of minutes the infusion is to run}}$$

References

Joint Formulary Committee (BNF) (2008) *British National Formulary (55)*. London: British Medical Association and Royal Pharmaceutical Society of Great Britain.

Lister S (2008) *Drug Administration General Principles*. In Doughty L and Lister S (eds) *The Royal Marsden Hospital Manual of Clinical Nursing Procedures* 7th edition. Oxford: Wiley-Blackwell Publishing.

National Institute for Health and Clinical Excellence (NICE) (2006) *Nutrition support for adults (CG32)*. London: National Institute for Health and Clinical Excellence. Available at: online http://www.nice.org.uk/nicemedia/pdf/CG032NICEguideline.pdf (accessed march 2009).

Royal College of Nursing (RCN) (2005) *Standards for Infusion Therapy*. London: Royal College of Nursing.

Case study 9.1

A 74–year-old woman is transferred from a residential home and admitted to the hospital with a diagnosis of right-upper-lobe pneumonia. She has a past medical history of lung cancer, hypertension, depression and anxiety disorder. Her observations are: B/P 150/86 mmHg; P 90 bpm; R 30 resps/min; T 38.3 °C. Her current medications include the following:

+ IV fluids: glucose 5% sodium chloride 0.45% 1000 mL 8 hourly
+ Azithromycin (Zithromax) 500 mg IV daily
+ EnsurePlus $\frac{3}{4}$ strength 800 mL via PEG to run from 0100 to 0800 daily
+ Alprazolam 0.5 mg via PEG 3 times a day (t.i.d)
+ Sertraline (Lustral) 50 mg by mouth (PO) at bedtime
+ Losartan potassium (Cozaar) 25 mg via PEG daily
+ Fluconazole 200 mg, oral suspension, via PEG immediately (stat), then 100 mg daily for 7 days
+ Docusate sodium 100 mg, oral suspension, via PEG twice daily (b.i.d.)
+ Furosemide (Lasix) 40 mg, oral suspenßsion via PEG twice daily (b.i.d.)
+ Paracetamol 1 g, oral suspension, via PEG 4 hourly prn if temperature above 38 °C

Read the labels in Figure 9.13, when necessary, to answer the following questions.

1. What is the rate of flow for the IV solution in mL per hour?
2. What is the rate of flow for the IV in drops/min? The drop factor rate is 15 drops/mL
3. The IV infusion was started at 1900 h (7pm). When will it be completed?
4. What is the amount of glucose and sodium chloride in the IV solution?
5. The directions printed on the azithromycin IV bag label read '500 mg in glucose 100 mL, infuse via pump over 60 minutes.' What is the pump setting in mL/h?
6. EnsurePlus is available in 250 mL cans.
   (a) How many cans will you need to prepare the strength prescribed?
   (b) Calculate the rate of flow in mL/h.

(a)
Fluconazole
For oral suspension
10 mg/mL

(b)
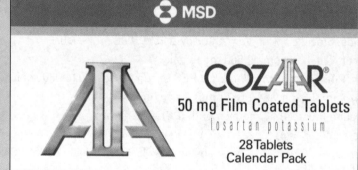

(c)
MSD

COZAAR®
50 mg Film Coated Tablets
losartan potassium
28 Tablets
Calendar Pack

(d)
Furosemide
Oral solution
10 mg per mL
Protect from light
Discard opened bottle after 90 days

(e)
Alprazolam
Oral solution
1 mg per mL
Protect from light
Discard 90 day after opening

Figure 9.13 Drug labels for Case Study 9.1

((b) Reprinted with permission, courtesy of Pfizer Ltd; (c) From Merck Sharp & Dohme Ltd, reproduced with permission)

7. How many millilitres of alprazolam will you administer?

8. How many millilitres of fluconazole will you prepare for the stat dose?

9. The label on the docusate sodium reads 60 mg/15 mL. How many millilitres contain the prescribed dose?

Practice sets

The answers to *Try these for practice and Exercises* appear in Appendix A at the end of the book.

Try these for practice

Test your comprehension after reading the chapter.

1. The prescriber orders *500 mL 5% glucose IV for 8 hours*. Calculate the flow rate in drops/min when the drop factor is 10 drops per millilitre. _____

2. The prescriber orders *1000 mL 0.9% NaCl IV over 8 hours*. The flow rate is 31 drops per minute. When the nurse assessed the infusion, 425 mL had infused in 4 hours. Calculate the new flow rate in drops/min if the drop factor is 15 drops per millilitre. _____

3. The prescriber orders *500 mL 5% glucose IV over 4 hours*. Calculate the flow rate in millilitres per hour. _____

4. An IV of glucose 4% saline 0.18% is infusing at a rate of 27 drops per minute. The drop factor is 15 drops/mL. How many millilitres per hour is the patient receiving? _____

5. Prescription: *Fresubin 400 mL over 6 hours via PEG*. Determine the pump setting in mL/h. _____

Exercises

Reinforce your understanding in class or at home.

1. The physician prescribes *750 mL of NaCl (0.9%) IV for 8 hours*. Calculate the flow rate in drops per minute. The drop factor is 10 drops = 1 mL.

   _____

2. The patient is to receive *375 mL of Ringer's Lactate over 3 hours*. Set the rate on the infusion pump in millilitres per hour.

   _____

3. The patient is prescribed *Ensure 50 mL per hour via feeding tube*. The drop factor is 10 drops per millilitre. Calculate the flow rate in drops per minute.

   _____

4. Prescription reads *1000 mL glucose to infuse at 125 mL/h*. The tubing is calibrated at 15 drops/mL. How long will this infusion take to finish?

   _____

5. A patient is to receive *500 mL glucose 4% saline 0.18% IV in 3 hours*. Calculate the flow rate in microdrops per minute. The giving set tubing is calibrate at 60 drops/mL.

   _____

6. The prescription reads *1500 mL glucose IV over 12 hours*. The drop factor is 20 drops/mL.

   (a) Find the flow rate in drops/min for this infusion.

   (b) If after 3 hours 1200 mL remain to be infused, how must the flow rate be adjusted so that the infusion will finish on time?

   (c) If the clinical area has a policy that flow rate adjustments must not exceed 25% of the original rate, is the adjustment required above in part (b) within the guidelines or does it fall outside the guidelines?

---

7. Prescription reads *750 mL Ringer's Lactate IV in 8 hours*. Calculate the flow rate in drops per minute if the drop factor is 15 drops/mL.

---

8. An IV infusion of 750 mL Ringer's Lactate began at noon (12.00). It has been infusing at the rate of 125 mL/h. At what time is it scheduled to finish?

---

9. A patient has an order for a total parenteral nutrition (TPN) solution 1000 mL in 24 hours. At what rate in mL/h should the pump be set?

---

10. An IV is infusing at 90 mL/h. The IV tubing has a drop factor of 20 drops/mL. Calculate the flow rate in drops/min.

---

11. Order: *1000 mL normal saline IV over 6 hours*. Calculate and set the flow rate in mL/h for the electronic controller.

---

12. Calculate the infusion time for an IV of 500 mL that is ordered to run at 40 mL/h.

---

13. The order reads *750 mL of normal saline IV. Infuse over a 24 h period*. Set the flow rate on the infusion pump in millilitres per hour.

---

14. An IV of 800 mL is to infuse over 8 hours at the rate of 20 drops/min. After 4 hours and 45 minutes, only 300 mL had infused. Recalculate the flow rate in drops/min. The set calibration is 15 drops/mL.

---

15. An IV solution is infusing at 32 microdrops per minute. How many millilitres of this solution will the patient receive in 6 hours?

Chapter 10

Calculating flow rates for intravenous medications

After completing this chapter, you will be able to

1. Describe intravenous medication administration.
2. Calculate the flow rate of intravenous solutions based on the amount of drug per minute or per hour.
3. Determine the amount of drug a patient will receive IV per minute or per hour.
4. Calculate IV flow rates based on body weight.
5. Calculate IV flow rates based on body surface area.
6. Calculate the infusion time of an IV solution.
7. Calculate the rate of flow for a medication requiring titration.

This chapter extends the discussion of intravenous infusions to include administration of intravenous medications. You will also learn how to calculate the flow rates for IVs based on body weight or body surface area (BSA.)

Diagnostic questions

Before commencing this chapter try to answer the following questions. Compare your answers with those in Appendix A.

1. Convert 60 mL per hour to mLs per minute
2. Convert 25 mL per minute to L per hour
3. A patient is to receive one dose of a drug at 5 mcg per kilogram body weight. He weighs 80 kg. How much of the drug should he have?
4. Convert 40 mg per minute to mg per hour.
5. A patient is receiving 900 mg of a drug over 90 minutes. How much of this drug would she have received after 1 hour?

Intravenous administration of medications

Intravenous administration of medications provides rapid access to a patient's circulatory system, thereby presenting potential hazards. Errors in medication, dose or dosage strength can prove fatal. Therefore, *caution must be taken in the calculation, preparation and administration of IV medications*.

Typically, a **primary** IV line provides continuous fluid to the patient. **Secondary** lines can be attached to the primary line at injection ports, and these lines are often used to deliver *continuous* or *intermittent* medication intravenously. With intermittent secondary infusions, the bags generally hold 50–250 mL of fluid containing dissolved medication and usually require 20–60 minutes to infuse. Like a primary line, a secondary infusion may use a manually controlled gravity system or an electronic pump. A **heplock**, or **saline lock**, is an infusion luerlock port attached to an indwelling needle or cannula in a peripheral vein. Intermittent IV infusions can be administered through these ports via IV lines connected to these ports. An **IV bolus** is a direct injection of medication either into the heplock/saline lock or directly into the vein.

Syringe pumps can also be used for intermittent infusions. A syringe with the medication is inserted into the pump. The medication is delivered at a set rate over a short period of time.

A **volume-control** set is a small container, called a **burette**, that is connected to the IV line. Burettes are often used in paediatric or elderly care, where accurate volume control is critical. The danger of overdose is limited because of the small volume of solution in the burette. Burettes will be discussed in Chapter 11.

Practice point

An IV bolus dose generally involves medications administered over a short period of time. Be sure to check and verify the need for the drug, route, concentration, dose, expiration date and clarity of the solution. It is also essential to check and verify the rate of injection with the package insert. Some medications (e.g. adenosine) require very rapid administration, whereas others (e.g. verapamil) are administered more slowly. Do not forget to observe the patient for signs of reactions also.

Secondary intravenous infusion lines

Patients can receive a medication through a port in an existing IV line. This is called a secondary *intravenous infusion line* (Figure 10.1). The medication is in a secondary bag. Notice in Figure 10.1 that the secondary bag is higher than the primary bag so that the pressure in the secondary line will be greater than the pressure in the primary line. Do stop the primary infusion to avoid back flow into this line (RCN, 2005). Once the secondary infusion is completed, the primary line begins to flow. Do check the types of infusion sets used in the clinical area and the procedure; some are connected via a luerlock connector and may need vigilance as the primary line will need to be restarted when the secondary infusion has completed.

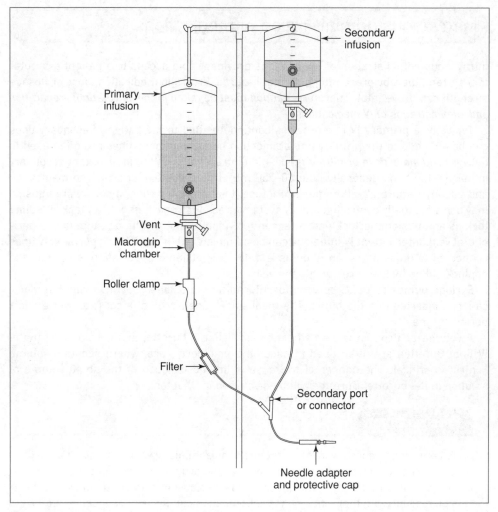

Figure 10.1 Primary and secondary infusion setup.

A typical IV prescription might read: *cimetidine 300 mg 6 hourly in 50 mL normal saline infuse over 30 min*. This is an order for an IV secondary infusion in which 300 mg of the drug cimetidine diluted in 50 mL of a normal saline solution must infuse in 30 minutes. So, the patient receives 300 mg of cimetidine in 30 minutes via a secondary line, and this dose is repeated every 6 hours. (See Figure 10.2)

Stop and think

According to the RCN Infusions (2005) guidelines you should stop the primary infusion whilst letting the secondary infusion infuse and be careful of 'backwash', thus giving a bolus of the drug later when the primary infusion is recommenced.

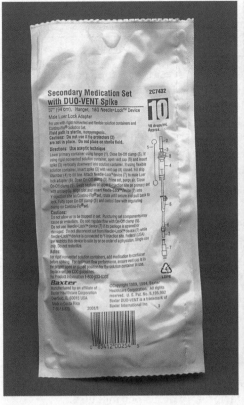
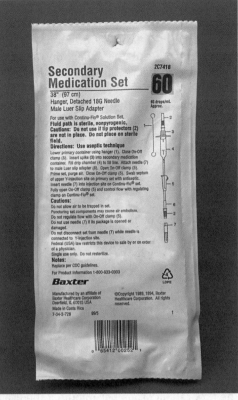

(a)   (b)

Figure 10.2 Packages of secondary IV tubing

(Baxter Healthcare/Photo by Al Dodge, Images provided courtesy of Baxter Healthcare Corporation)

Example 10.1

The prescriber orders: *Cefotazidime 1 g IV 4 hourly.* The package insert information is as follows: 'Add 50 mL sterile water to the bag of cefotazidime 1 g and infuse in 30 min'. The tubing is labelled 20 drops per millilitre. Calculate the flow rate in drops per minute for this antibiotic.

The patient receives 50 mL in 30 min. You want to change this flow rate from mL per minute to an equivalent flow rate in drops per minute:

$$\frac{50 \text{ mL}}{30 \text{ min}} \longrightarrow \frac{? \text{ drops}}{\text{min}}$$

Using the drop factor of 20 drops/mL, you can do this on one line as follows:

$$\frac{50 \text{ mL}}{30 \text{ min}} \times \frac{20 \text{ drops}}{1 \text{ mL}} = \frac{100 \text{ drops}}{3 \text{ min}} = 33.3 \frac{\text{drops}}{\text{min}}$$

So, the flow rate is *33 drops per minute*.

Example 10.2

The order is *Cefotaxime 1 g IV 6 hourly in 50 mL over 30 min*. Read the label for the premixed Cefotaxime in Figure 10.3 and find the drip rate if the drop factor is 10 drops/mL. The package insert indicates that the Cefotaxime should be infused in 30 minutes. The label states: '1 g in 50

> Cefotaxime 1 g
> IV Single Dose container
> Vial 50 mL contains 1 g

Figure 10.3 Drug label for cefotaxime

mL. This entire solution must be infused in 30 minutes'. You want to change the flow rate from 50 mL per 30 minutes to an equivalent flow rate in drops per minute:

$$\frac{50 \text{ mL}}{30 \text{ min}} \longrightarrow \frac{? \text{ drops}}{\text{min}}$$

Using the drop factor of 10 drops/mL, you can do this on one line as follows:

$$\frac{50 \text{ mL}}{30 \text{ min}} \times \frac{10 \text{ drops}}{\text{mL}} = \frac{50 \text{ drops}}{3 \text{ min}} = 16.67 \frac{\text{drops}}{\text{min}}$$

So, the flow rate is *17 drops per minute*.

Example 10.3

The prescription reads *1000 mL 5% glucose with 1000 mg of a drug at 1 mg/min*. Calculate the flow rate in drops per minute if the drop factor is 15 drops per millilitre.

In this example, the prescriber has specified the amount of solution and its strength (1000 mL of 5% glucose containing 1000 mg of the drug) and also the rate at which the patient receives the drug (1 mg/min). This 'flow rate' is not the usual volume per time (mL/h or drops/min), but it is in terms of weight of drug per time (mg/min).

Given flow rate:	1 mg/min (notice that a flow rate always has 'time' in the denominator)
Known equivalences:	1000 mg/1000 mL (strength)
	15 drop/mL (drop factor)
Flow rate you want to find:	? drops/min

You want to convert the flow rate from milligrams per minute to an equivalent flow rate in drops per minute:

$$1 \frac{\text{mg}}{\text{mL}} \longrightarrow \frac{\text{drops}}{\text{min}}$$

You want to cancel mg. To do this you must use a unit fraction containing mg in the denominator. Using the strength, this fraction will be $\dfrac{1000 \text{ mL}}{1000 \text{ mg}}$:

$$1 \frac{\text{mg}}{\text{min}} \times \frac{1000 \text{ mL}}{1000 \text{ mg}} = \frac{? \text{ drops}}{\text{min}}$$

Now, on the left side mL is in the numerator, and it must be cancelled. This will require a unit fraction with mL in the denominator. Using the drop factor, this fraction will be $\dfrac{15 \text{ drops}}{\text{mL}}$. Now cancel and multiply the numbers:

$$\frac{1 \ \cancel{mg}}{1 \ min} \times \frac{\cancel{1000} \ \cancel{mL}}{\cancel{1000} \ \cancel{mg}} \times \frac{15 \text{ drops}}{1 \ \cancel{mL}} = \frac{15 \text{ drops}}{min}$$

So, you would administer *15 drops per minute*.

Stop and think

Always note how drugs are prescribed, e.g. mg or units. Do not forget any relevant metric equivalents so: 1 unit = 1000 milliunits (mU). This is always a factor of a thousand which could lead to an over- or under-dose of a drug.

Example 10.4

The prescriber writes a prescription for 1000 mL of 5% glucose with 10 units of a drug. Your patient must receive 30 mU of this drug per minute. Calculate the flow rate in microdrops per minute.

Given flow rate:	30 mU/min (notice that a flow rate always has 'time' in the denominator)
Known equivalences:	10 units/1000 mL (strength)
	60 drops/mL (standard microdrop drop factor)
	1 unit = 1000 mU
Flow rate you want to find:	? mcdrops/min

You want to change the flow rate from milliunits per minute to microdrops per minute.

You want to cancel mU. To do this you must use a unit fraction containing mU in the denominator. Using the equivalence 1 mU = 1000 units, this fraction will be $\dfrac{1 \text{ unit}}{1000 \text{ mU}}$.

Now, on the left side unit is in the numerator, and it must be cancelled. This will require a unit fraction with unit in the denominator. Using the strength, this fraction will be $\dfrac{1000 \text{ mL}}{10 \text{ units}}$.

Now, on the left side mL is in the numerator, and it must be cancelled. This will require a unit fraction with mL in the denominator. Using the drop factor, this fraction will be mcdrop $\dfrac{60 \text{ mcdrop}}{\text{mL}}$. Now, cancel and multiply the numbers:

$$\frac{30 \ \cancel{mU}}{min} \times \frac{1 \ \cancel{unit}}{\cancel{1000} \ \cancel{mU}} \times \frac{\cancel{1000} \ \cancel{mL}}{10 \ \cancel{units}} \times \frac{60 \text{ mcdrop}}{\cancel{mL}} = 180 \text{ mcdrop/min}$$

So, you will administer *180 mcdrops/min*.

Example 10.5

Calculate the flow rate in millilitres per hour if the prescription reads *Add 10 000 units of heparin to 1000 mL 5% glucose IV*. Your patient is to receive 1250 units of this anti-coagulant per hour via an infusion pump.

You want to change the flow rate from units per hour to millilitres per hour:

$$\frac{1250 \text{ units}}{1 \text{ h}} \longrightarrow ? \frac{\text{mL}}{\text{h}}$$

Using the strength of the solution (10 000 units/1000 mL) you do this on one line as follows:

$$\frac{1250 \text{ units}}{1 \text{ h}} \times \frac{1000 \text{ mL}}{10\ 000 \text{ units}} = \frac{1250 \text{ mL}}{10 \text{ h}} = 125 \frac{\text{mL}}{\text{h}}$$

So, your patient will receive 125 mL per hour.

Double check this – you could use the old formula:

$$\frac{\text{drug dose}}{\text{drug available}} \times \text{volume it is in}$$

or

$$\frac{1250 \text{ units}}{10\ 000} \times 1000 \text{ mL} = \underline{125.1 \text{ mL/h}}$$

In Examples 10.6 and 10.7 you are given the flow rate in millilitres per hour, and you need to determine the amount of medication the patient will receive in a given amount of time.

Example 10.6

Calculate the number of units of Regular insulin a patient is receiving per hour if the order is *500 mL normal saline with 300 units of Regular insulin and it is infusing at the rate of 12.5 mL per hour via the pump*.

You want to convert the flow rate from mL per hour to units per hour:

$$\frac{12.5 \text{ mL}}{\text{h}} \longrightarrow ? \frac{\text{units}}{\text{h}}$$

Using the strength of the solution (300 units/500 mL) you do this in one line as follows:

$$\frac{12.5 \text{ mL}}{\text{h}} \times \frac{300 \text{ units}}{500 \text{ mL}} = \frac{37.5 \text{ units}}{5 \text{ h}} \quad \text{or} \quad 7.5 \frac{\text{units}}{\text{h}}$$

So, the patient is receiving *7.5 units per hour*.

Example 10.7

Your patient is receiving an IV of 1000 mL of NaCL (normal saline) with 1000 mg of the bronchodilator drug aminophylline. The flow rate is 50 mL/h. How many milligrams per hour is your patient receiving?

You want to convert the flow rate from millilitres per hour to milligrams per hour:

$$\frac{50 \text{ mL}}{1 \text{ h}} \longrightarrow ? \frac{\text{mg}}{\text{h}}$$

Using the strength of the solution (1000 mg/1000 mL) you do this on one line as follows:

$$\frac{50 \text{ mL}}{1 \text{ h}} \times \frac{1000 \text{ mg}}{1000 \text{ mL}} = 50 \frac{\text{mg}}{\text{h}}$$

So, your patient is receiving *50 mg per hour*.

Stop and think

Use estimations to guide the 'area' of where your calculations might be. In Example 10.7: 1 mg = 1 mL, thus 50 mg/h = 50 mL/h. Some may not be so straightforward, but estimate first, then calculate and always double check.

Calculating flow rates based on body weight

In Chapter 5 you calculated dosages based on *body weight alone*. Suppose a patient weighing 100 kg is to receive a drug at the rate of *2 micrograms per kilogram* (2 mcg/kg). You could convert the single unit of measurement (kg) into the single unit of measurement (mcg), and the patient would receive 200 mcg of the drug as the following calculation shows:

$$100 \text{ kg} \times \frac{2 \text{ mcg}}{\text{kg}} = 200 \text{ mcg}$$

In this chapter you will see that some IV medications are not only prescribed based on the patient's body weight, but the amount of drug the patient receives also depends on time. For example, a prescription might indicate that a drug is to be administered at the rate of *2 micrograms per kilogram per minute* (2 mcg/kg/min). This means that *each minute* the patient is to receive 2 mcg of the drug for every kilogram of body weight. Therefore, the amount of medication the patient receives is based on *both body weight and time*. For calculation purposes this new type of rate (compound rate) is written as

$$\frac{2 \text{ mcg}}{\text{kg} \times \text{min}}$$

Imagine that a patient weighing 100 kg is receiving a drug at the rate of 2 mcg/kg/min. If you multiply the weight of this patient (a single unit of measurement) by the compound rate, you obtain a rate which depends only on *time* as follows:

$$100 \text{ kg} \times \frac{2 \text{ mcg}}{\text{kg} \times \text{min}} = \frac{200 \text{ mcg}}{\text{min}}$$

So, the patient is receiving the drug at the rate of 200 mcg/min.

Titrating medications

Sometimes medications must be **titrated**. That is, the dose of the medication must be adjusted until the desired therapeutic effect (e.g. blood pressure maintenance) is achieved. This is often seen within high-dependency situations, e.g. intensive care or high-dependency units. Example 10.8 includes a drug that is titrated.

Example 10.8

Prescription: *dopamine 2 mcg/kg/min IV infusion, titrate to maintain systolic blood pressure above 90, increase by 5 mcg/kg/min every 10–30 minutes. Maximum dose 20 mcg/kg/min. Monitor BP and HR every 2–5 minutes during titration*. The label on the 500 mL medication bag states: '800 mcg/mL', and the patient weighs 79.5 kg.

1. How many mcg/min of dopamine should the patient receive initially?
2. Calculate the initial pump setting in mL/h.

1. You want to convert the weight of the patient (79.5 kg) to micrograms of dopamine per minute:

$$79.5 \text{ kg} \longrightarrow \frac{\text{mcg}}{\text{min}}$$

You can do this on one line as follows:

$$79.5 \text{ kg} \times \frac{2 \text{ mcg}}{\text{kg}} \times \text{min} = 159 \frac{\text{mcg}}{\text{min}}$$

So, initially the patient will receive *159 mcg/min*.

2. Now, convert $159 \frac{\text{mcg}}{\text{min}}$ to $\frac{\text{mL}}{\text{h}}$. Using the strength of the solution (800 mcg/mL) and

   1 h = 60 min you can do this on one line as follows:

$$\frac{159 \text{ mcg}}{\text{min}} \times \frac{1 \text{ mL}}{800 \text{ mcg}} \times \frac{60 \text{ min}}{\text{h}} = 11.96 \frac{\text{mL}}{\text{h}}$$

So, the pump would initially be set at *12 mL/h*.

Practice point

Drugs that are titrated are powerful drugs and must follow the local policy and protocol. Therefore, you must know the local policy. If in doubt do ask, be safe.

Calculating flow rates based on body surface area

As you know, certain medications are prescribed based on body surface area (BSA). Chapter 5 discussed how to determine BSA, and you may find it helpful to revisit this before proceeding with the next exercise. Examples 10.9–10.11 show how to calculate flow rates for this type of medication order (BSA).

Example 10.9

The order is *100 mg/m² IV infusion in 50 mL normal saline (NaCL)*. The patient has a BSA of 1.55 m². The drug package information indicates that the infusion should be given over 30 minutes. The label on the vial indicates that the strength of the reconstituted drug is 38 mg/mL.

1. How many mg of the drug would the patient receive?
2. How many mL of the drug would you need to take from the vial?
3. What is the total volume (in mL) to be infused?
4. What is the flow rate in mL/h?
5. If the drop factor is 10 drops/mL, what is the rate of flow in drops/min?

1. First make an estimation – the dose is 100 mg/m² and the patient's BSA is 1.55 m². Therefore, the patient will need *more than 100 mg but less than 200 mg*.

   You want to change the size of the patient (in m²) to the number of milligrams of the drug.

   $$1.55 \text{ m}^2 \longrightarrow ? \text{ mg}$$

   $$1.55 \text{ m}^2 \times \frac{100 \text{ mg}}{\text{m}^2} = 155 \text{ mg}$$

   So, the patient would receive *155 mg* of the drug.

2. You want to convert the amount of drug (in mg) to the volume of drug (in mL).

   $$155 \text{ mg} \longrightarrow ? \text{ mL}$$

   The label indicates that the strength of the reconstituted the drug is 38 mg/mL.

   $$155 \text{ mg} \times \frac{1 \text{ mL}}{38 \text{ mg}} = 4.1 \text{ mL}$$

Since your patient should receive 4.1 mL of the drug, 4.1 mL should be withdrawn from the vial.

3. Since the 4.1 mL of the drug must be added to the 50 mL bag, the total volume to be infused will be $(50 + 4.1) = 54.1\ mL$.

4. Since the entire volume must infuse in 30 minutes ($\frac{1}{2}$ hour), you need to simplify and convert this to mL/h. The flow rate, in millilitres per hour, is therefore:

$$\frac{54.1\ \text{mL}}{\frac{1}{2}\ \text{h}} = 108.2\ \frac{\text{mL}}{\text{h}}$$

5. Since the drop factor is 10 drops = 1 mL, the flow rate found in part (d) can be converted to drops/min as follows:

$$\frac{108.2\ \cancel{\text{mL}}}{\cancel{\text{h}}} \times \frac{10\ \text{drops}}{\cancel{\text{mL}}} \times \frac{1\ \cancel{\text{h}}}{60\ \text{min}} = 18.03\ \frac{\text{drops}}{\text{min}}$$

So, the flow rate, in drops per minute, is *18 drops/min*.

Stop and think

Be clear that you know the local policy concerning IV medications that are reconstituted for administration. Determine whether in the calculations, the total volume to be infused must include the volume of the added reconstituted medication. For example, in Example 10.9 if the volume of the reconstituted drug added to the IV bag (4.1 mL) had been ignored in the calculations, the answer to part (d) would have been (50 mL/$\frac{1}{2}$ h) = 100 mL/h instead of 108.2 mL/h. This may mean incorrect infusion rate and reduced amount of the drug administered to the patient.

Example 10.10

Prescription: *Irinotecan (antineoplastic drug) 125 mg/m^2 IV infusion in 250 mL of normal saline (NaCL) over 90 minutes once weekly for 4 weeks*. The patient has a BSA of 1.67 m^2. Read the label for this antineoplastic drug in Figure 10.4 and determine the pump setting in millilitres per hour.

First, change the size of the patient (BSA) to the number of millilitres needed to be taken from the Campto vial:

$$1.67\ \text{m}^2 \longrightarrow ?\ \text{mL}$$

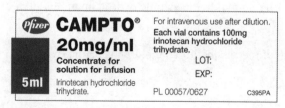

Figure 10.4 Drug label for Campto

(Reproduced with permission, courtesy of Pfizer Ltd)

From the order, you need to use 125 mg/m²; and from the label, the concentration of the irinotecan is 100 mg/5 mL:

$$1.67 \, \text{m}^2 \times \frac{125 \, \text{mg}}{\text{m}^2} \times \frac{5 \, \text{mL}}{100 \, \text{mg}} = 10.4 \, \text{mL}$$

So, 10.4 mL is taken from the irinotecan vial and is added to the 250 mL bag. This means that the total volume of the infusion is (250 + 10.4) = 260.4 mL, and the patient would receive 260.4 mL of irinotecan in 90 minutes.

Now, change the flow rate of $\dfrac{260.4 \, \text{mL}}{90 \, \text{min}}$ to mL/h:

$$\frac{260.4 \, \text{mL}}{90 \, \text{min}} \times \frac{60 \, \text{min}}{\text{h}} = 173.6 \, \text{mL/h}$$

So, the pump is set at *174 mL/h.*

Example 10.11

A patient who weighs 55 kg is receiving a medication at the rate of 30 mL/h. The concentration of the medication is 400 mg in 500 mL of glucose 5%. The recommended dose range for the drug is 2–5 mcg/kg/min. Is the patient receiving a safe dose?

Method 1
Convert the safe dose range of 2–5 mcg/kg/min to mL (of the drug)/hour.

First, use the minimum recommended dose (2 mcg/kg/h) and start with the weight of the patient to determine how many mL/h the patient should minimally receive as follows:

$$55 \, \text{kg} \times \frac{2 \, \text{mcg}}{\text{kg} \times \text{min}} \times \frac{60 \, \text{min}}{\text{h}} \times \frac{1 \, \text{mg}}{1000 \, \text{mcg}} \times \frac{500 \, \text{mL}}{400 \, \text{mg}} = 8.3 \frac{\text{mL}}{\text{h}} \quad \text{min}$$

Now, use the maximum recommended dose (5 mcg/kg/h) and start with the weight of the patient to determine how many mL/h the patient should maximally receive as follows:

$$55 \, \text{kg} \times \frac{5 \, \text{mcg}}{\text{kg} \times \text{min}} \times \frac{60 \, \text{min}}{\text{h}} \times \frac{1 \, \text{mg}}{1000 \, \text{mcg}} \times \frac{500 \, \text{mL}}{400 \, \text{mg}} = 20.6 \frac{\text{mL}}{\text{h}} \quad \text{max}$$

So, the safe dose range for this patient is 8.3–20.6 mL/h. Since the patient is receiving 30 mL/h, the patient is not receiving a safe dose, but is receiving an overdose.

Method 2
Convert the 30 mL/h, which the patient is receiving, to mcg/kg/min and then compare this to the safe dose range of 2–5 mcg/kg/min.

This may be a mathematically more sophisticated approach, but it requires fewer calculations. Realise that what you are looking for, mcg/kg/min, is in the form of amount of drug/weight of patient/time. An amount of drug (30 mL) is being administered to a 55 kg patient over a period of time (1 hour). So, the patient is receiving 30 mL/55 kg/1 h.

You want to change 30 mL/55 kg/1 h to mcg/kg/min, which can be done in one line as follows:

$$\frac{30 \text{ mL}}{55 \text{ kg} \times 1 \text{ h}} \times \frac{1 \text{ h}}{60 \text{ min}} \times \frac{400 \text{ mg}}{500 \text{ mL}} \times \frac{1000 \text{ mcg}}{1 \text{ mg}} = 7.3 \frac{\text{mcg}}{\text{kg} \times \text{min}}$$

The safe dose range for this patient is 2–5 mcg/kg/min, since the patient is receiving 7.3 mcg/kg/min, the patient is not receiving a safe dose, but an overdose.

Practice point

Whenever your calculations indicate that the prescribed dose is not within the safe range, you should check the prescription with the prescriber. Some drugs are highy toxic and may be fatal, too much vitamin C may not be dangerous but too much morphine could be. You are responsible for giving the drug.

Summary

In this chapter, the IV medication administration process was discussed. IV infusions and IV bolus administrations were described, and prescriptions based on body weight and body surface area were demonstrated and practised.

+ A secondary line is sometimes used and follows the same care as a primary line (changing, etc.). Always close the primary infusion when the secondary one is in progress.

+ IV bolus medications can be injected into a heplock/saline lock or directly into the vein.

+ The IV bag that is hung highest will infuse first; thus the rates of primary and secondary infusions relying on gravity need to be checked regularly.

+ A prescription containing *mg/kg/min* means that each minute, the patient must receive the stated number of milligrams of medication for each kilogram of the patient's body weight.

+ For calculation purposes and to assist in understanding write mg/kg/min as $\dfrac{\text{mg}}{\text{kg} \times \text{min}}$.

+ When calculating rates of flow of infusions based on body weight or BSA, start with the patient's size, as measured by weight or BSA.

+ When looking for *mg/kg/min*, start with the amount of *drug/weight/time*.

+ When titrating medications, the dose is adjusted and constantly monitored until the desired therapeutic effect is achieved.

+ Always double check calculations.

Reference

Royal College of Nursing (RCN) (2005) *Standards for Infusion Therapy*. London: Royal College of Nursing.

Case study 10.1

A middle aged man is admitted to your clinical area with a diagnosis of deep vein thrombosis (DVT). He has pain in his right calf muscle area and on examination it looks inflamed and is tender. He feels well generally apart from the pain in his right leg. His height is 1.8 m and weight 78 kg. His observations are: T 37 °C, P 88/min; R 18/min; B/P 140/80 mmHg. He is to be monitored on the ward for signs of deterioration and to commence anticoagulation therapy.

His prescription reads:

+ Increase oral fluids – minimum of 2 L/day
+ Heparin 5000 units IV immediately (stat)
+ Heparin 18 units/kg/hour by continuous IV infusion
+ Warfarin 3 mg PO daily to be rechecked after 5 days and amended to ensure the INR (International Normalised Ratio – ratio of a patient's prothrombin time to a normal (control) sample and an indicator of clotting) is within therapeutic range (2.0–2.5, tested by blood sample).
+ Paracetamol 1 g for pain 6 hourly PRN

1. Calculate the stat dose of heparin for this patient. The vial indicates 25,000 U/mL.

2. Determine if the heparin infusion is in the safe dose range – the normal heparinising range is between 20 000 and 40 000 units per day.

3. Warfarin is supplied in 1 mg and 2 mg tablets. How many and of what type would you give to the patient for one daily dose?

4. The patient finds it difficult to swallow tablets but requests paracetamol for pain. The paracetamol is dispensed as an oral suspension of paracetamol 250 mg/5 mL. How many mLs would you give to your patient?

5. If this patient drinks three cups of tea (150 mL each) and two cans of cola (330 mL each), how much more fluid does he have to take to achieve his minimum intake?

Practice sets

The answers to *Try these for practice and Exercises* appear in Appendix A at the end of the book.

Try these for practice

Test your comprehension after reading the chapter.

1. Prescription: *Cimetidine 300 mg IV infusion 6 hourly in 50 mL NaCl infused over 30 min.* The drop factor is 15 drops/mL. Find the flow rate in drops/min. _____

2. The prescription is for a continuous infusion of theophylline at a rate of 25 mg/h. It is diluted in 5% glucose to produce a concentration of 500 mg per 500 mL. Determine the rate of the infusion in mL/h. _____

3. A 500 mL 5% glucose solution with 2 g of procainamide HCl is infusing at 15 mL/h via a volumetric pump. How many mg/h is the patient receiving? _____

4. Prescription: *Dobutamine 250 mg in 250 mL of 5% glucose at 3.5 mcg/kg/min.* Determine the flow rate in mcdrops/min for a patient who weighs 54.5 kg. _____

5. A patient is receiving heparin 1200 units/hour. The directions for the infusion are: 'add 25 000 units of heparin in 250 mL of solution.' Determine the flow rate in mL/h. _____

Exercises

Reinforce your understanding in class or at home.

1. A maintenance dose of norepinephrine bitartrate 2 mcg/min IV infusion has been ordered to infuse using an 8 mg in 250 mL of 5% glucose solution. What is the pump setting in mL/h?

2. The patient is receiving lidocaine at 40 mL/h. The concentration of the medication is 1 g per 500 mL of IV fluid. How many mg/min is the patient receiving?

3. Prescription: *Dopamine 400 mg in 250 mL glucose 5% at 3 mcg/kg/min IV infusion.* Calculate the flow rate in mL/h for a patient who weighs 91 kg.

4. A drug is ordered 180 mg/m^2 in 500 mL normal saline 0.90% to infuse over 90 minutes. What is the flow rate in mL/h?

5. How long will a 550 mL bag of intralipids take to infuse at the rate of 25 mL/h?

6. The patient is receiving heparin at 1000 units/hour. The IV has been prepared with 24 000 units of heparin per litre. Find the flow rate in mL/h.

7. Prescription: *Humulin S 50 units in 500 mL NaCl infuse at 1 mL/min IV pump.* How many units per hour is the patient receiving?

8. An IV infusion of 50 mL is to infuse in 30 minutes. After 15 minutes, the IV bag contains 40 mL. If the drop factor is 20 drops/mL, recalculate the flow rate in drops/min.

9. The patient is receiving *nitroprusside 50 mg in 250 mL of 5% glucose* for hypertension. The rate of flow is 20 mL/h. If the patient weighs 75 kg, determine the dosage in micrograms/kilogram/minute the patient is receiving. (Hint: do this in stages.)

10. Prescription: *Warfarin sodium 4 mg IV bolus stat to be administered over 1 minute.* The available 5 mg of warfarin is in a vial with directions that state to dilute with 2 mL of sterile water:

    (a) How many mg will the patient receive?

    (b) How many mL will you administer?

    (c) How many mL/min will be infused?

11. The patient is to receive *Methyldopa 500 mg IV infusion dissolved in 100 mL of IV fluid over 60 minutes.* If the drop factor is 15 drops/mL, determine the rate of flow in drops/min.

12. The patient is to receive *isoproterenol at a rate of 4 mcg/min.* The concentration of the isoproterenol is 2 mg per 500 mL of IV fluid. Find the pump setting in mL/h.

13. The patient is receiving *aminophylline at the rate of 20 mL/h.* The concentration of the medication is 500 mg/1000 mL of IV fluid. How many mg/h is the patient receiving?

14. *Nipride 3 mcg/kg/min* has been ordered for a patient who weighs 82 kg. The solution has a strength of 50 mg in 250 mL of 5% glucose. Calculate the flow rate in mL/h.

15. A medication is ordered at 75 mg/m^2 IV bolus. The patient has BSA of 2.33 m^2. How many millitres of the medication will be administered if the vial is labelled 50 mg/mL?

Chapter 11

Calculating paediatric dosages

Learning outcomes

After completing this chapter, you will be able to

1. Determine if a paediatric dose is within the safe dose range.
2. Calculate paediatric oral and parenteral dosages based on body weight.
3. Calculate paediatric oral and parenteral dosages based on body surface area.
4. Calculate daily fluid maintenance.

Because the metabolism and body mass of children are different from those of adults, paediatric medication dosages are usually less than adult dosages.

Paediatric nurses and health professionals appreciate that children are not merely small adults and thus it is insufficient to give smaller doses of drugs. As there is a lack of licensed medications in suitable formulations for children, extra care is needed with checking the drugs prescribed and the doses to be administered as often this depends upon body mass and age. The recent European Union regulation on paediatric medicines will address some of the issues of medicines adapted and licensed for children (MHRA 2008), and this will eventually ease some of the complex calculation burdens. Paediatric formularies are available (for example BNFC, 2007). Hutton (2005) identifies that accuracy with calculations for paediatric patients is paramount as they cannot compensate physiologically and the potential for harm is thus enormous. In this chapter you will learn and practise the principles and techniques behind the calculation of paediatric doses and appreciate the implications for other vulnerable groups, e.g. the elderly.

Diagnostic questions

Before commencing this chapter try to answer the following questions, then compare your answers with those in Appendix A.

1. A child is to have a drug dose of 5 mg per kg body weight. This child is given 5 mg is this correct?

2. Measure out 250 mg of an antibiotic. The dose in the bottle reads: 125 mg in 5 mLs. How many mLs do you give?

3. What is 40 mL multiplied by 20?

4. What is $0.4 \times 2.4 \times 12$?

5. What is 0.75×0.30?

Safe paediatric drug dosages

At the present time, the most accurate method of determining an appropriate paediatric dose is based on body weight. Body surface area is also used, especially in paediatric oncology and critical care. You must be able to determine whether the amount of a pre-scribed paediatric dosage is within the safe range. In order to do this, you must compare the child's ordered dosage to the recommended safe dosage as found in a reputable drug resource. First, determine the recommended dose or dosage range found on the summary of product characteristics (SPC) leaflet, in the hospital formulary, in the *British National Formulary for Children (BNFC)* or in a pharmacology text.

Administration of oral and parenteral medications

When prescribing medications for the paediatric population, the oral route is preferred. However, if a child cannot swallow, or the medication is ineffective when given orally, the parenteral route is used.

Oral medications

The developmental age of the child must be taken into consideration when determining the device to administer oral medication. For example, an older child may be able to swallow a pill or drink a liquid medication from a cup. An oral syringe, calibrated dropper or measuring spoon may be selected when giving medication to an infant or younger child (see Figures 11.1 and 11.2).

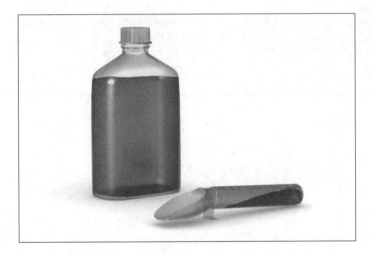

Figure 11.1 Measuring spoon

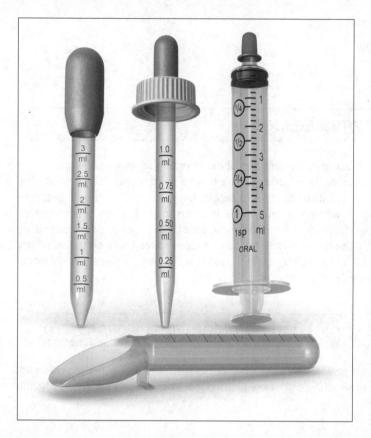

Figure 11.2 Liquid medicine administration

Parenteral medications

Subcutaneous or intramuscular routes may be necessary, depending on the type of medication to be administered. Because of the small muscle mass of children, usually not more than 1 mL is injected.

Calculating drug dosages by body weight

Drug manufacturers sometimes recommend a dosage based on the weight of the patient. Body weight or body mass is most frequently used when prescribing drugs for infants and children.

Example 11.1

The prescription states *erythromycin 10 mg/kg PO 8 hourly*. Read the label in Figure 11.3. The child weighs 40 kg. How many millilitres of the drug will you administer to this child?

You want to convert the body weight to the dose in millilitres:

$$40 \text{ kg} \rightarrow ? \text{ mL}$$

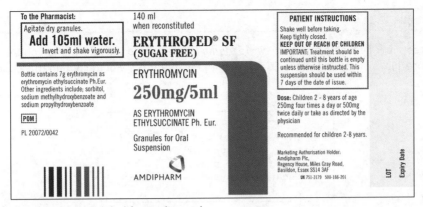

Figure 11.3 Drug label for Erythroped
(Reproduced with permission of Amdipharm Plc)

Do this on one line as follows:

$$40 \text{ kg} \times \frac{? \text{ mg}}{? \text{ kg}} \times \frac{? \text{ mL}}{? \text{ mg}} = ? \text{ mL}$$

Because the prescription is 10 mg/kg, the first unit fraction is $\dfrac{10 \text{ mg}}{1 \text{ kg}}$.

Because the strength is 250 mg/5 mL, the second unit fraction is $\dfrac{5 \text{ mL}}{250 \text{ mg}}$.

You cancel the kilograms and milligrams and obtain the dose in millilitres:

$$40 \, \cancel{\text{kg}} \times \frac{10 \, \cancel{\text{mg}}}{\cancel{\text{kg}}} \times \frac{5 \text{ mL}}{250 \, \cancel{\text{mg}}} = 8 \text{ mL}$$

So, the child should receive *8 mL* of erythromycin.

Example 11.2

The prescription is for *cefuroxime 15 mg/kg PO 12 hourly*. How many milligrams of this antibiotic would you administer to a child who weights 25 kg?

You want to convert body weight to a dose in milligrams:

$$25 \text{ kg} \rightarrow ? \text{ mg}$$

$$25 \text{ kg} \times \frac{? \text{ mg}}{? \text{ kg}} = ? \text{ mg}$$

Because the order is 15 mg/kg the unit fraction is $\dfrac{15 \text{ mg}}{\text{kg}}$. You cancel the kilograms and obtain the dose in milligrams:

$$25 \, \cancel{\text{kg}} \times \frac{15 \text{ mg}}{\cancel{\text{kg}}} = 375 \text{ mg}$$

So, the child would receive *375 mg* of cefuroxime.

Example 11.3

The prescriber requests *azithromycin 15 mg/kg PO stat.* Read the information on the label in Figure 11.4. The child weighs 18 kg. How many millilitres would contain this dose?

```
          Azithromycin
        Oral suspension
        200 mg per 5 mL
   Discard 10 days after opening
```

Figure 11.4 Drug label for azithromycin

You want to convert the body weight to a dose in millilitres:

$$18 \text{ kg} \rightarrow ? \text{ mL}$$

Do this on one line as follows:

$$18 \text{ kg} \times \frac{? \text{ mg}}{? \text{ kg}} \times \frac{? \text{ mL}}{? \text{ mg}} = ? \text{ mL}$$

Because the order is 15 mg/kg, the first unit fraction is $\dfrac{15 \text{ mg}}{\text{kg}}$.

Because the strength is 200 mg per 5 mL the second unit fraction is $\dfrac{5 \text{ mL}}{200 \text{ mg}}$. You cancel the milligrams and obtain the dose in millilitres:

$$18 \, \cancel{\text{kg}} \times \frac{15 \, \cancel{\text{mg}}}{\cancel{\text{kg}}} \times \frac{5 \text{ mL}}{200 \, \cancel{\text{mg}}} = 6.75 \text{ mL}$$

So, you would prepare 6.7 mL of azithromycin. *Note:* paediatric doses are generally rounded down.

Example 11.4

The recommended dosage for neonates receiving Ceftazidime is 30 mg/kg IM every 12 hours. If an infant weighs 2600 g how many milligrams of Ceftazidime would the neonate receive in one day?

On estimation you see that the child weights more than 1 kg, in fact more than 2 kg but less than 3 kg; thus, the dose will be more than 60 mg but less than 90 mg. You want to convert the body weight to a dose in milligrams:

$$2600 \text{ g (body weight)} \rightarrow ? \text{ mg (drug)}$$

Do this on one line as follows:

$$2600 \text{ g} \times \frac{? \text{ kg}}{? \text{ g}} \times \frac{? \text{ mg}}{? \text{ kg}} = ? \text{ mg}$$

Because 1 kg = 1000 g, the first unit fraction is $\frac{1 \text{ kg}}{1000 \text{ g}}$.

Because the recommended dosage is 30 mg/kg, the second equivalent fraction is $\frac{30 \text{ mg}}{1 \text{ kg}}$.

$$2600 \text{ g} \times \frac{1 \text{ kg}}{1000 \text{ g}} \times \frac{30 \text{ mg}}{\text{kg}} = 78 \text{ mg per dose}$$

Since the neonate receives two doses per day, the total daily dose is *156 mg.*

Example 11.5

The prescription reads *morphine sulphate 0.3 mg IM stat.* The recommended dose is 0.01 milligram per kilogram. Is the ordered dose safe for a child who weighs 31 kg?

You want to convert the body weight to the recommended dose in milligrams:

$$31 \text{ kg} \rightarrow ? \text{ mg}$$

$$31 \text{ kg} \times \frac{? \text{ mg}}{? \text{ kg}} = ? \text{ mg}$$

Because the recommended dose is 0.01 mg/kg, the unit fraction is $\frac{0.01 \text{ mg}}{\text{kg}}$. You cancel the kilograms and obtain the dose in milligrams:

$$31 \text{ kg} \times \frac{0.01 \text{ mg}}{1 \text{ kg}} = 0.31 \text{ mg}$$

The recommended dose is 0.31 mg, whereas the ordered dose is 0.3 mg. So, 0.3 mg is a safe dose of morphine sulphate for this child.

Stop and think

Always make an estimation before doing the calculation – this ensures you have an idea of the dose. Always think whether it is grams of milligrams, where is the decimal point, etc. – always double check calculations. Many clinical areas require two nurses to check calculations and doses, and this is especially important in paediatrics.

Calculating drug dosages by body surface area

Drug manufacturers may recommend a paediatric dosage based on body surface area (BSA). A nomogram is generally used to determine body surface area (see Figure 11.5) which is read using height and weight.

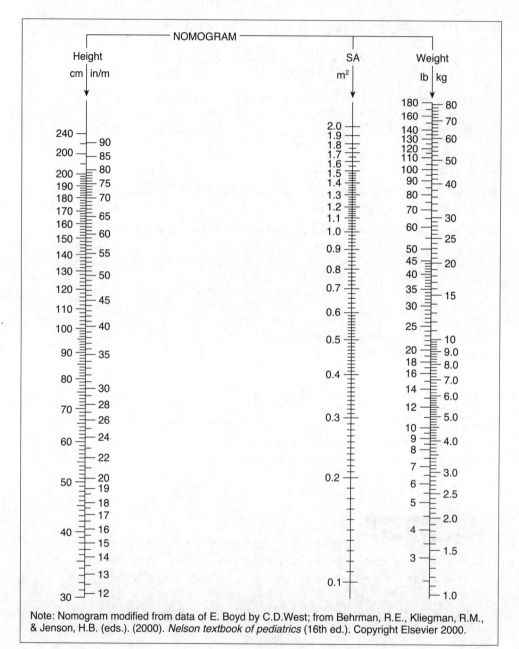

Note: Nomogram modified from data of E. Boyd by C.D.West; from Behrman, R.E., Kliegman, R.M., & Jenson, H.B. (eds.). (2000). *Nelson textbook of pediatrics* (16th ed.). Copyright Elsevier 2000.

Figure 11.5 Nomogram

Example 11.6

If a child has a BSA of 0.75 m², and the medication order is for actinomycin-D 0.5 mg/m² daily for 5 days IV bolus, what dose (in milligrams) of this antineoplastic (cancer) drug should the child receive?

On estimation you know the child is less than 1 m² so the dose is less than 0.5 mg. You want to convert the body surface area to a dose in milligrams:

$$0.75 \text{ m}^2 \rightarrow ? \text{ mg}$$

$$0.75 \text{ m}^2 \times \frac{? \text{ mg}}{? \text{ m}^2} = ? \text{ mg}$$

Because the order is 0.5 mg/m², the unit fraction is $\dfrac{0.5 \text{ mg}}{\text{m}^2}$. You cancel the square metres and obtain the dose in milligrams:

$$\frac{0.75 \cancel{\text{m}^2}}{1} \times \frac{0.5 \text{ mg}}{1 \cancel{\text{m}^2}} = 0.375 \text{ mg}$$

So, *0.37 mg* of actinomycin-D should be administered.

Practice point

Some children can look smaller or larger for their age; thus it is important to use medication doses based on body surface area.

Example 11.7

Diazepam 3.75 mg was prescribed for a child with status epilepticus. The package information SPC says that the recommended dose is 0.2–0.5 mg/kg IV bolus slowly every 2–5 minutes up to a maximum of 5 mg. The child weighs 33 lbs, and the label on the vial reads 5 mg/mL.

1. Is the ordered dose within the safe range?

2. How many millilitres would you administer?

1. You want to convert the body weight in *pounds* to *kilograms*; then convert the body weight in *kilograms* to a recommended dose in *milligrams*:

$$33 \text{ lb (body weight)} \rightarrow ? \text{ kg (body weight)} \rightarrow ? \text{ mg (drug)}$$

Do this on one line as follows:

$$33 \text{ lb} \times \frac{? \text{ kg}}{? \text{ lb}} \times \frac{? \text{ mg}}{? \text{ kg}} = ? \text{ mg}$$

Because 1 kg = 2.2 lb, the unit fraction is $\dfrac{1 \text{ kg}}{2.2 \text{ lb}}$.

Because the recommended dosage is 0.2–0.5 mg/kg per day, you need to find the minimum and the maximum recommended doses in milligrams for this patient. Use the unit fractions $\dfrac{0.2 \text{ mg}}{\text{kg}}$ and $\dfrac{0.5 \text{ mg}}{\text{kg}}$:

$$\frac{33 \text{ lb}}{1} \times \frac{1 \text{ kg}}{2.2 \text{ lb}} \times \frac{0.2 \text{ mg}}{\text{kg}} = 3 \text{ mg} \quad 3 \text{ mg is the minimum dose}$$

$$\frac{33 \text{ lb}}{1} \times \frac{1 \text{ kg}}{2.2 \text{ lb}} \times \frac{0.5 \text{ mg}}{\text{kg}} = 7.5 \text{ mg} \quad 7.5 \text{ mĺg is the maximum dose}$$

The safe dose range for this patient is 3–7.5 mg.

Because the ordered dose of 3.75 mg is between 3 mg and 7.5 mg, it is a safe dose.

2. You want to convert the prescribed dosage in milligrams to the liquid daily dose in millilitres:

$$3.75 \text{ mg (drug)} \rightarrow \text{? mL (drug)}$$

Do this on one line as follows:

$$3.75 \text{ mg} \times \frac{\text{? mL}}{\text{? mg}} = \text{? mL}$$

Because the vial label says that 5 mg/mL, the unit fraction is $\dfrac{1 \text{ mL}}{5 \text{ mg}}$:

$$\frac{3.75 \text{ mg}}{1} \times \frac{1 \text{ mL}}{5 \text{ mg}} = 0.75 \text{ mL}$$

Always remember the mantra: amount you want divided by amount available, multiplied by the volume.

So, you would administer *0.75 mL* of the Diazepam IV bolus slowly.

Practice point

Know the local policy concerning the procedure and type of fluid to flush the intravenous lines or burette. Be aware of drug left in the tubing as insufficient drug may be given or the residual drug may be given too rapidly via flushing.

Administration of intravenous medications using a volume control chamber

Paediatric intravenous medications are frequently administered using a **volume control chamber (VCC)**. In order to avoid fluid overload, a VCC (burette, Volutrol, Buretrol, Soluset) is often used when administering paediatric intravenous fluids (see Figure 11.6).

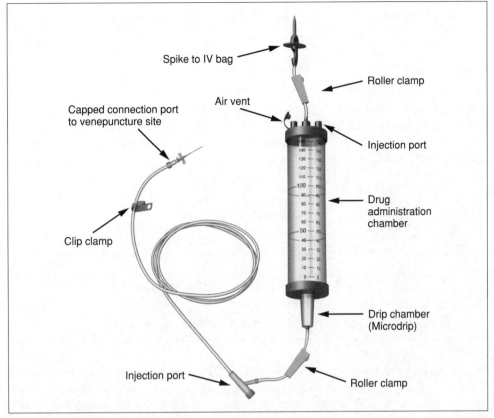

Figure 11.6 Volume control chamber

A VCC is calibrated in 1 mL increments and has a capacity of 100–150 mL. It can be used as a primary or secondary line. Pumps are normally used to deliver fluids and drugs to children; however, it is necessary to check on the progress of fluids to ensure they are being administered correctly.

Example 11.8

The doctor prescribes *gentamicin 25 mg IV 8 hourly* for a child who weighs 20 kg. The medication is supplied in 20 mg vials with a strength of 10 mg/mL.

1. How many millilitres would you withdraw from the vials?
2. Using a burette, how many millilitres of IV solution do you need to add to obtain the recommended concentration of 2 mg/mL?

1. You want to convert the order of 25 mg to mL:

$$25 \text{ mg} \rightarrow ? \text{ mL}$$

$$25 \text{ mg} \times \frac{? \text{ mL}}{? \text{ mg}} = ? \text{ mL}$$

Because the vial label says that the strength is 10 mg/mL, the unit fraction is $\dfrac{1\ mL}{10\ mg}$:

$$\frac{25\ \cancel{mg}}{1} \times \frac{1\ mL}{10\ \cancel{mg}} = 2.5\ mL$$

So, you would withdraw *2.5 mL* from the vial.

2. The 2.5 mL (containing 25 mg of gentamicin) taken from the vial is added to the burette and it then needs to be further diluted to a concentration of 2 mg/mL.

You must convert the 25 mg of gentamicin in the burette to millilitres of solution of strength 2 mg/mL:

$$25\ mg \rightarrow ?\ mL$$

$$25\ mg \times \frac{?\ mL}{?\ mg} = ?\ mL$$

Because the recommended concentration is 2 mg/mL, the unit fraction is $\dfrac{1\ mL}{2\ mg}$:

$$\frac{25\ \cancel{mg}}{1} \times \frac{1\ mL}{2\ \cancel{mg}} = 12.5\ mL\ \text{of solution in the VCC}$$

So, *10 mL* (12.5–2.5 mL) of IV solution should be added to the burette.

In summary, in Example 11.8, you would add the *2.5 mL from the vial of gentamicin* to the top injection port of a volume control chamber (burette) (see Figure 11.6) and then add an additional *10 mL of IV solution* from the bag to obtain the *12.5 mL*, which will contain the recommended *safe medication concentration*.

Example 11.9

Prescription: *chloramphenicol 500 mg in 100 mL of glucose 5% IV infusion 6 hourly.* The recommended dose is 50–75 mg/kg/day in divided doses given every 6 hours. The child weighs 34.6 kg. Is the prescription in the safe dose range?

Method 1
Convert both the safe dose range and the prescribed dose to mg/day.

First, use the minimum safe dose (50 mg/kg/day) to determine how many mg/day the patient should minimally receive as follows:

$$34.6\ \cancel{kg} \times \frac{50\ mg}{\cancel{kg} \times day} = 1730\ \frac{mg}{day}\ \text{min}$$

Now, use the maximum safe dose (75 mg/kg/day) to determine how many mg/day the patient should maximally receive as follows:

$$34.6\ \cancel{kg} \times \frac{75\ mg}{\cancel{kg} \times day} = 2595\ \frac{mg}{day}\ \text{max}$$

So, the safe dose range for this patient is 1730–2595 mg/day.

The ordered dose is 500 mg every 6 hours. Convert this to mg/day as follows:

$$\frac{500 \text{ mg}}{6 \text{ h}} \times \frac{24 \text{ h}}{\text{day}} = 2000 \frac{\text{mg}}{\text{day}}$$

The ordered dose is equivalent to 2000 mg/day. This is within the safe dose range of 1730–2595 mg/day and the patient is receiving a safe dose.

Method 2

Convert the ordered dose of 500 mg every 6 hours, to mg/kg/day. Then compare this to the safe dose range of 50–75 mg/kg/day. This may be a mathematically more sophisticated approach, but it requires fewer calculations.

Realise that what you are looking for, mg/kg/day, is in the form of amount of drug/weight over patient/time. An amount of drug (500 mg) is prescribed for a (34.6 kg) patient over a period of time (6 hours). So, the order is 500 mg/34.6 kg/6 h.

You want to change this to mg/kg/day, which can be done in one line as follows:

$$\frac{500 \text{ mg}}{34.6 \text{ kg} \times \overset{1}{6 \text{ h}}} \times \frac{\overset{4}{24 \text{ h}}}{\text{day}} = 57.8 \frac{\text{mg}}{\text{kg} \times \text{day}}$$

The ordered dose is equivalent to 57.8 mg/kg/day. This is within the safe dose range of 50–75 mg/kg/day.

Stop and think

Do check the ranges of drug doses in both methods (daily and patient weight). Ensure that you use the same units of measurement, e.g. grams or milligrams, not a mixture which can be confusing and potentially dangerous.

Calculating daily fluid maintenance

The administration of paediatric intravenous medications requires careful and exact calculations and procedures. Infants and severely ill children are not able to tolerate extreme levels of hydration and are quite susceptible to dehydration, fluid overload and drug overdose. Therefore, you must closely monitor the amount of fluid a child receives. The fluid a child requires over a 24-hour period is referred to as **daily maintenance fluid needs**. Daily maintenance fluid includes both oral and parenteral fluids. The amount of maintenance fluid required depends on the weight of the patient (see the formula in Table 11.1). The daily maintenance fluid does not include body fluid losses through vomiting, diarrhoea or fever. Additional fluids referred to as **replacement fluids** (usually Lactated Ringer's or 0.9% NaCl) are utilised to replace fluid losses and are based on each child's condition (e.g. if 20 mL are lost, then 20 mL of replacement fluids are usually added to the daily maintenance).

Table 11.1 Maintenance fluid requirements

Paediatric daily fluid maintenance formula	
0–10 kg	4 ml/kg/hr
10–20 kg	40 ml/hr + 2 ml/kg/hr above 10 kg
>20 kg	60 ml/hr + 1 ml/kg/hr above 20 kg

(Formula of Holliday and Segar, APAGBI, 2007)

Example 11.10

If the prescription is *half maintenance* for a child who weighs 25 kg, at what rate should the pump be set in mL/h?

As the child is 25 kg, using the calculation in Table 11.1 the child is 20 kg plus 5 kg. Thus they should receive 60 ml/h (for 20 kg weight) plus 5×1 ml/kg/h. So this is:

$$60 \text{ mL/h} + 5 \text{ mL/h} = 65 \text{ mL/h}$$

As this is half maintenance dose (50%) half of 65 mL = 32.5 mL. So, the pump would be set at *33 mL/h*.

Summary

In this chapter you calculated oral and parenteral dosages for paediatric patients. Some dosages were based on body weight or BSA. Daily fluid maintenance needs were calculated. You also determined whether ordered dosages were in the safe dose range.

+ Taking shortcuts in paediatric medication administration can be fatal.

+ Check to see if the prescription is in the safe dose range.

+ Consult a reliable source when in doubt about a paediatric drug prescription.

+ Question the prescription or check your calculations if the prescribed dose differs from the manufacturer's recommended dose.

+ Amounts of medication used for children are small: no more than 1 mL should be given IM, and IV bags of no more than 500 mL should be commenced.

+ Paediatric dosages are generally rounded down.

+ Because accuracy is crucial in paediatric infusions, electronic control devices or volume control chambers should always be used.

+ For a volume control chamber, a flush is always used to clear the tubing after the medication is infused.

+ Know the local policy regarding the inclusion of medication volume as part of the total infusion volume.

+ Daily fluid maintenance depends on the weight of the child and includes both oral and parenteral fluids.

References

Association of Paediatric Anaesthetists of Great Britain and Ireland (APAGBI) (2007) *APA Consensus Guidelines on perioperative Fluid Management in Children v.1.1*. London: Association of Paediatric Anaesthetists of Great Britain and Ireland. Available at: http://www.rcoa.ac.uk/apagbi/docs/Perioperative_Fluid_Management_2007.pdf (accessed March 2008).

British National Formulary for Children (BNFC) (2007) *British National Formulary for Children*. London: British Medical Association, the Royal Pharmaceutical Society of Great Britain, the Royal College of Paediatrics and Child Health, and the Neonatal and Paediatric Pharmacists Group.

Hutton M (2005) Paediatric Nursing Calculation Skills. *Paediatric Nursing* **17**(2): 1–17.

Medicines and Healthcare Products Regulatory Agency (MHRA) (2008) *Medicines for children*. London: Medicines and Healthcare Products Regulatory Agency. Available at: http://www.mhra.gov.uk/Howweregulate/Medicines/Medicinesforchildren/index.htm (accessed March 2009).

Case study 11.1

A 4-year-old girl is admitted to the hospital with a diagnosis of pneumonia. Her parents say that she has been very irritable, has had a chronic cough, decreased appetite, and diarrhoea for almost a week. On examination, the child has laboured breathing with the crackles in the right upper lobe (RUL) of the lung. She is also mildly cyanosed. She is small in stature for a child of her age (96 cm tall) and underweight (14 kg). She is allergic to milk products. Her observations are: T 37.6 °C; BP 88/64 mmHg; P 100/min; R 26/min. Throat swab was positive for Group A streptococcus. Her care and prescription include the following:

+ Bed rest
+ Diet as tolerated, encourage oral fluids
+ Fluids 1800 mL/m^2 day
+ Salbutamol 1 mg with 2 mL saline 8 hourly via nebuliser
+ Benzylpenicillin 425 mg in 50 mL glucose 5% IV 6 hourly
+ Vitamin ADEK 2 mL once daily in A.M.

1. Calculate the child's 24-hour fluid requirement.
2. The recommended dose for benzylpenicillin is 100 mg/kg/day divided in 4 equal doses (to be given every 6 hours). Is the ordered dose safe?
3. The benzylpenicillin is available in 600 mg vial. Calculate the setting in mL/h on the infusion pump to administer the benzylpenicillin over 30 minutes.
4. If the usual dose range of salbutamol is 0.1–0.15 mg/kg per dose, is the salbutamol dose safe for this child?

Practice sets

The answers to *Try these for practice*, *Exercises* and *Cumulative review exercises* appear in Appendix A at the end of the book.

Try these for practice

Test your comprehension after reading the chapter.

1. The following order has been given for a child who weighs 45 kg: *Humulin S insulin 0.1 unit/kg subcutaneously b.i.d. before breakfast and dinner.* How many units will this child receive of this insulin in 24 h? _____

2. Order: *Zidovudine 90 mg IV 6 hourly.* The patient is a two-year-old child with BSA of 0.62 m². If the recommended safe dose range is 100–180 mg/m² 6 hourly, is the prescribed dose safe? _____

3. The order is *amoxicillin 250 mg PO.* The label reads 125 mg/5 mL. How many millilitres would you administer? _____

4. Read the information on the label in Figure 11.7. How many millilitres of codeine would you administer to a child who weighs 40 kg when the prescription is 0.3 mg/kg PO 4 hourly. _____

```
          Codeine phosphate
           Oral solution
           15 mg per 5 mL
```

Figure 11.7 Drug label for codeine

5. The prescription reads *IV glucose 4%, NaCl 0.18% (glucose-saline)* at maintenance and one half for a 42 kg child. How many mL/h does the child need? _____

Exercises

Reinforce your understanding in class or at home.

1. The prescriber orders *gentamicin 50 mg IV 8 hourly* for a child who weighs 18 kg. The recommended dosage is 6–7.5 mg/kg/day divided in three equal doses. Is the prescribed dose within the safe range?

2. The prescription reads *vancomycin 10 mg/kg 12 hourly, IV* for a neonate who weighs 4000 g. What is the dose in milligrams?

3. The prescriber orders *methotrexate 2.9 mg PO weekly* for a child who is 106 cm tall and weighs 23 kg. The package insert states that the recommended dosage is 7.5–30 mg/m² every 1–2 weeks. Is the order a safe dose?

4. Prescription: *paracetamol 10 mg/kg PO 4 hourly prn* for a child who weighs 32 kg. How many milligrams will you administer?

5. A manufacturer recommends giving 350 mg/m^2/day to a maximum of 450 mg/m^2/day for a drug. A child has a BSA of 1.2 m^2. Calculate the safe dose range (in milligrams per day) for this child.

6. Prescription: *cefuroxime suspension 30 mg/kg/day 8 hourly*. The child weighs 35 kg. The label reads 187 mg/mL. How many millilitres will you administer?

7. Prescription: *1000 mL glucose 5% infuse at 65 mL/h*. The drop factor is 60 microdrops/mL. Calculate the infusion rate in microdrops per minute.

8. Prescription: *ranitidine 30 mg IV 8 hourly*. The patient weighs 23 kg. The package SPC insert states that the recommended dose in paediatric patients is for a total dose of 2–4 mg/kg/day, to be divided and administered every 6–8 hours, up to a maximum of 50 mg per dose. Is the prescribed dose safe?

9. Prescription: *IV glucose 4%, NaCl 0.18% (glucose saline)*.

   (a) The child weighs 25 kg. If the child is NPO (to take nothing orally), what is the daily IV fluid maintenance?

   (b) What is the rate of flow in mL/h?

10. A child has a BSA of 0.82 m^2. The recommended dose of a drug is 2 million units/m^2. How many units will you administer?

11. Order: *cefotamine sodium (Claforan) 1.2 g IV 8 hourly*. The safe dose range for the solution concentration is 20–60 mg/mL to infuse over 15–30 minutes. What is the minimal amount of IV fluid needed to safely dilute this dosage? [Hint: The minimal amount of IV fluid is the maximal safe concentration.]

12. Order: *Zidovudine (Retrovir) 160 mg/m^2 8 hourly PO*. The child has a BSA of 1.1 m^2. Read the label in Figure 11.8. How many millilitres will you prepare?

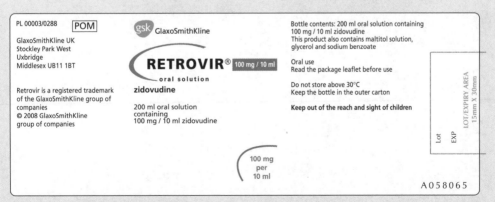

Figure 11.8 Drug label for Retrovir

(Reproduced with the permission of GlaxoSmithKline)

13. Prescription indicates: *erythromycin 125 mg PO 4 hourly*. The child weighs 14.5 kg. The usual dosage is 30–50 mg/kg/day in equally divided doses. The label reads: 'erythromycin 200 mg/5 mL'.

    (a) Is the prescribed dose safe?

    (b) How many mg would you administer?

14. Prescription: *vancomycin 40 mg/kg/day IV 6 hourly to infuse over 90 minutes in 200 mL normal saline*. The child weighs 41 kg. The Vancomycin has a concentration of 50 mg/mL. What will you set the pump at in mL/h?

15. A medication of 100 mg in 1 mL is diluted up to 15 mL and administered IV bolus over 20 minutes. How many mg/min is the patient receiving?

Cumulative review exercises

Review your mastery of Chapters 9–11.

32. You have a sodium chloride solution with a concentration of 0.45%. How many milligrams of sodium chloride are in 1 mL?

_____

33. The order reads *Compleat-B 480 mL via PEG every 12 h*. At how many mL/h will you set the pump?

_____

34. A patient is prescribed 2500 mL of 20% glucose to infuse over 16 hours. Set the rate on the infusion pump at millilitres per hour.

_____

35. An IV of 1000 mL of 5% glucose is to infuse at a rate of 30 drops per minute for 10 hours. After 4 hours, the patient had received 600 mL. The drop factor is 15 drops per millilitre. Recalculate the flow rate in drops/min.

_____

36. Calculate the BSA of a patient who is 178 cm and weighs 90 kg (hint: look at the calculation in Chapter 5).

_____

37. The patient has a BSA of 1.6 m^2. The prescription is 0.8 mg/m^2. The drug is supplied in 1.2 mg capsules. How many capsules will you prepare?

_____

38. An intravenous solution is infusing at 80 microdrops per minute. How many millilitres per hour is the patient receiving? _____

39. The patient must receive 1 500 000 units of penicillin IM, and the vial contains 20 000 000 units (in powdered form). The directions on the vial are: 'Add 38.7 mL to the vial; 1 mL = 500 000 units'. How many millilitres will equal 1 500 000 units?

_____

40. A patient must receive 0.5 mg of scopolamine IM, a parasympathetic antagonist. The label on the ampoule reads 0.3 mg/mL. How many millilitres will you administer to this patient? _____

41. The prescription is *Cefuroxime 200 mg PO every 12 hours for 10 days*. The bottle is labelled 100 mg/5 mL. How many millilitres of this antibiotic will you give your patient? _____

42. If you have a vial labelled 120 mg/mL, how many millilitres would equal 1.2 g?

_____

43. How many milligrams PO of ethambutol HCI (Myambutal), an antituberculosis drug, would you administer if the prescribed dose is 15 milligrams per kilogram and the child weighs 35 kg? _____

44. How many units of regular insulin subcutaneously would you prepare for a child who weighs 30 kg if the prescription is 1 unit per kilogram? _____

45. The prescription reads *cefuroxime 8 mg/kg PO once daily*:

(a) How many milligrams of this antibiotic would you administer to a child whose weight is 25 kg?

(b) Each tablet contains 0.2 g. How many tablets will you administer? _____

46. The order reads *50 units of Lente insulin subcutaneously before breakfast*. The vial is labelled 100 units per millilitre. How many units would you administer to the patient? _____

47. The prescriber has prescribed 10 million units of penicillin G IV every 12 hours. The 20-million-unit vial of powder has these instructions: 'add 40 mL of sterile water'. How many millilitres equal 10 000 000 units? _____

48. The order is *300 mg of ranitidine PO*. The label indicates that each capsule contains 150 mg.

(a) How many capsules equal the prescribed dose? _____

(b) Calculate the dose in grams. _____

49. The prescriber writes *900 mL of 5% glucose IV in 5 h*. Calculate the flow rate in drops per minute when the drop factor is 20 drops per millilitre. _____

50. A patient is receiving 1000 mL 5% glucose at 17 drops/min IV. The infusion began at 21.00 h (9:00 P.M.). At what time will this solution be completed? The drop factor is 15 drops per millilitre. _____

Comprehensive self-tests

Answers to *Comprehensive self-tests* 1–4 can be found in Appendix A at the back of the book.

1. Calculate the dosage of calcium EDTA drug for a patient who has a body surface area (BSA) of 1.47 m². The recommended dose is 500 mg/m².

2. Kineret (anakinra) 100 mg subcutaneous daily has been prescribed for a patient with rheumatoid arthritis. The prefilled syringe is labeled 100 mg/mL. Calculate the dose in grams.

3. An IV of 1000 mL 5% glucose is infusing at a rate of 40 drops/min. How long will it take to finish if the drop factor is 20 drops/mL?

4. Calculate the number of grams of glucose in 250 mL of 5% glucose.

5. The prescriber ordered *Cordarone (amiodarone HCl) 400 mg PO b.d.* Each tablet contains 200 mg. How many tablets will you give the patient?

6. The prescriber ordered an antibiotic 1 g IV 12 hourly to infuse in 30 minutes. The label on the premixed IV bag reads: 'Antibiotic 50 mL, 50 mg/mL'.

   (a) Calculate the flow rate in millilitres per hour.

   (b) How many milligrams will the patient receive?

7. Your patient is to receive morphine sulphate 5 mg subcutaneously stat. The 20 mL multiple dose vial is labelled morphine 15 mg/mL. Calculate the dose and place an arrow on the syringe indicating the dose.

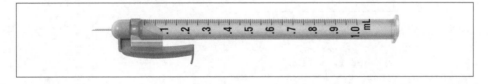

8. A prescriber orders a premixed solution of nitroglycerine 25 mg in 250 mL 5% glucose to be titrated at a rate of 5 mcg/min, increase every 5–10 min until pain subsides. The drug is to be infused via pump. How many mL/h will you set the pump to begin the infusion?

9. Prescription order: *Actrapid insulin 100 units in 100 mL normal saline, infuse at 0.1 unit/kg/h.* The patient weighs 68 kg. How many units per hour is the patient receiving?

10. The prescriber orders *Cefotaxime, 750 mg IM every 12 hours.* The 1 g vial of cefotaxime is in a powder form. The package leaflet states for IM injection, add 3 mL of sterile water for injection for an approximate volume of 3.4 mL containing 300 mg/mL. How many millilitres will you give the patient?

11. Prescription: *Lanoxin (digoxin) elixir 0.15 mg PO 12 hourly*. The child weighs 32 kg and the recommended maintenance dose is 7–10 mcg/kg/day.

    (a) What is the minimum daily maintenance dosage in mg/day?

    (b) What is the maximum daily maintenance dosage in mg/day?

    (c) Is the dose ordered safe?

12. *Doxycycline hyclate (Vibramycin) 4.4 mg/kg IV infusion daily* is ordered for a child who weighs 36 kg. The premixed IV solution bag is labelled: 'Doxocycline 200 mg/250 mL 5% Glucose to infuse in 4 hours'.

    (a) How many milligrams of Doxocycline must the patient receive?

    (b) How many mLs will the child receive?

13. The prescription reads *levofloxacin (Tavanic) 500 mg in 100 mL 5% glucose IV infusion daily for 14 days to infuse in 1 h*. Calculate the flow rate in drops per minute if the drop factor is 15 drops/mL.

14. Order: *Heparin 5000 units subcutaneous 12 hourly*. The multidose vial label reads 10 000 units/mL. How many millilitres will you give the patient?

15. Order: *10% glucose 1000 mL to infuse at 75 mL/h*. The drop factor is 20 drops/mL.

    (a) What is the rate of flow in $\dfrac{mL}{min}$?

    (b) How many drops per minute will you set the IV to infuse?

    (c) How long will it take for the infusion to be complete?

16. Calculate the total daily fluid maintenance for a child who weighs 45 kg.

17. Prescription order: *cephalexin (Keflex) oral suspension 50 mg/kg PO 6 hourly*. The label reads: '125 mg/5 mL'. The patient weighs 33 lbs. How many millilitres will you give over one day (4 doses)?

18. Read the label in Figure S.1.

    (a) How many milligrams of furosemide are in 1 mL?

    (b) How many millilitres of furosemide are in the bottle?

```
        Furosemide
       Oral solution
        10 mg per mL
      Protect from light
Discard opened bottle after 90 days
           60 mL
```

Figure S.1 Drug label for furosemide

19. The prescriber ordered *abciximab (ReoPro) 0.125 mcg/kg IV in 250 mL normal saline to be infused in 12 hours* for a patient who weighs 75 kg. The Abciximab label reads 2 mg/mL.

    (a) How many milligrams will the patient receive?

    (b) Calculate the flow rate in millilitres per hour.

Comprehensive self-test 2

1. A patient has an IV of 250 mL Ringers Lactate with 25 000 units of heparin infusing at 20 mL/h. How many units of heparin is the patient receiving each hour?

2. Prescription: *melphalan HCl (Alkeran) 16 mg/m² IV every 2 weeks for 4 doses. Infuse in 20 min*. The package leaflet states to rapidly inject 10 mL of supplied diluent into a 50 mg vial and shake vigorously until a clear solution results (5 mg/mL). The patient has a BSA of 1.2 m². You are assisting an experienced cancer nurse with this drug. Answer her questions:

    (a) How many milligrams contain the prescribed dose?

    (b) How many millilitres of melphalan will you add to 100 mL of normal saline?

3. A patient is receiving *ranitidine HCl (Zantac) 150 mg PO b.d.* The label reads; 150 mg tablets. How many tablets will the patient receive in 24 hours?

4. The prescription reads *Protamine sulphate 22 mg IV bolus over 10 min.*

    The label reads: '50 mg/5 mL. Dilute with 20 mL of normal saline or 5% glucose'.

    How many millilitres of protamine sulphate will you prepare?

5. The prescription reads: *gentamicin sulphate 9 mg IM 12 hourly*. The patient information leaflet states that the recommended dose for neonates is 2.5 mg/kg every 12–24 hours. The label on the vial reads: 'Paediatric Injectable Gentamycin 10 mg/mL'. The infant weighs 4.5 kg.

    (a) Is the dose safe?

    (b) How many millilitres will you give?

6. An IV of 5% glucose (1000 mL) is infusing at 50 mL/h. The infusion started at 13.00 h; what time will it finish?

7. The prescriber orders *phenytoin sodium (Dilantin) 250 mg/m²* in three divided doses for a child who has a BSA of 1.25 m². The bottle is labelled 125 mg/5 mL oral suspension. How many millilitres will you give for each dose?

8. The prescription reads *furosemide (Lasix) 20 mg IM stat.* The label reads: 40 mg/4 mL.

    (a) How many millilitres will you give the patient?

    (b) Place an arrow on the syringe that indicates the dose.

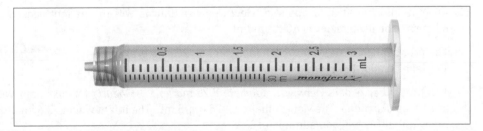

9. The recommended dose of Clindamycin paediatric oral solution is 8–25 mg/kg/day in three to four equally divided doses. A child weighs 27 kg.

    (a) Calculate the minimum safe daily dose.

    (b) Calculate the maximum safe daily dose.

10. Calculate how many grams of sodium chloride are in 250 mL of a 0.9% NaCl solution.

11. A patient has an IV infusing at 25 drops/min. How many mL/h is the patient receiving? The drop factor is 15 drops/mL.

12. Calculate the total daily volume and hourly IV flow rate for a 4.5 kg infant who is receiving maintenance fluids. (Hint: 4 mL/kg/h)

13. The prescription reads *nitroprusside sodium 50 mg in 250 mL 5% glucose infuse at 1 mL/h*. The recommended dosage range is 0.1–5 mcg/kg/min. The patient weighs 70 kg. Is this a safe dose?

14. Your patient has an IV of Actrapid insulin 50 units in 500 mL of normal saline infusing at 12 units per hour. Calculate the flow rate in mL/h.

15. Prescription: *ticarcillin disodium (Ticar) 1 g IM every 6 hours*. The package patient informa- tion leaflet states to reconstitute each 1 g vial with 2 mL of sterile water for injection. Each 2.5 mL = 1 g. How many millilitres will you administer?

16. The prescription states *docusate sodium (Docusol) syrup 100 mg via PEG t.i.d.* The label reads: 50 mg/15 mL. How many mL will you give?

17. Prescription: *theophylline 0.8 mg/kg/h IV via pump*. The premixed IV bag is labelled theophylline 800 mg in 250 mL 5% glucose. The patient weighs 84 kg. How many mL/h will you set the pump?

18. The nurse has prepared 7 mg of dexamethasone for IV administration. The label on the vial reads: 10 mg/mL. How many millilitres did the nurse prepare?

19. The prescription states *benzatropine mesilate 2 mg IM stat and then 1 mg IM daily*. The label reads: 2 mg/2 mL.

    (a) How many millilitres will you administer daily?

    (b) What size syringe will you use?

20. An IV of 250 mL 0.9% NaCl is infusing at 25 mL/h. The infusion began at 18.00 h. What time will it be completed?

Comprehensive self-test 3

1. An IV is infusing at 35 drops/min. How many millilitres will the patient receive in 6 hours? The drop factor is 10 drops/mL.

2. The prescription states *amoxicillin (Augmentin), 200 mg oral suspension PO 12 hourly*. The label reads: 125 mg/5 ml. How many millilitres will you administer?

3. The prescriber orders *neomycin sulphate 8.75 mg/kg PO 6 hourly* for an infant with infectious diarrhoea. The vial is labelled: 125 mg/5 mL. The infant weighs 3.6 kg. How many millilitres will you administer?

4. Prescription: *heparin 40 000 units in 1000 mL NaCl, infuse at 40 mL/h*: The normal heparinising range is 20 000–40 000 units every 24 hours. Calculate the units/h and determine if the dose is safe.

5. A prescriber orders *aluminum hydroxide 10 mL every 2 hours prn*. The label reads: 675 mg/5 mL. What is the maximum dose in milligrams that the patient may receive in 24 hours?

6. A patient is to receive 3500 units of heparin subcutaneously. The label reads: 10 000 units/mL. How many millilitres will you administer?

7. Prescription: *lamivudine (Epivir) oral solution 150 mg PO b.d.* The recommended safe dose is 4 mg/kg b.d. Is this a safe dose for a child who weighs 19 kg?

8. Prescription: *potassium chloride 40 mmol PO daily*. The label reads: 'potassium chloride 20 mmol per 15 mL'. How many millilitres will you administer?

9. Calculate the hourly IV flow rate and total daily IV fluid volume for a child who is NPO (taking nothing orally), weighs 6.8 kg, and is receiving maintenance fluids. (Hint: 4 mL/kg/h)

10. The prescription states *Actrapid insulin 24 units and Insulatard insulin 17 units subcutaneous before breakfast*. Draw an arrow on the syringe indicating the dose of each of the insulins.

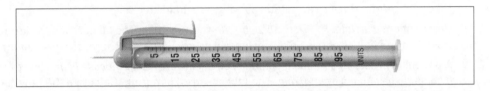

11. A patient who is 160 cm tall and weighs 60 kg is to receive *interferon alpha-2b (Intron A) 20 000 units/m²*. How many units contain this dose? (Hint: BSA to 2 decimal places.)

12. A patient is receiving an IV of 1000 mL of 5% glucose with 15 mmol of potassium chloride for 24 hours. Calculate the flow rate in mL/h. The drop factor is 10 drops/mL.

13. A patient is receiving TPN 1500 mL at a rate of 65 mL/h via pump. The infusion began at 06.00. What time will it be finished?

14. Prescription: *Ethambutol HCl 15 mg/kg PO daily*. The label reads: 400 mg tablets. How many tablets will you give the patient who weighs 80 kg?

15. A patient is receiving *Allopurinol 300 mg PO daily*. What is the total number of grams per day?

16. A patient has an IV of 0.9% sodium chloride infusing at 75 mL/h.

    The drop factor is 60 drops/mL. Calculate the flow rate in drops per minute.

17. Prescription: *Dexamethasone 1.5 mg PO daily*. The label reads: 0.75 mg tablets. How many tablets will you give?

18. Calculate the body surface area for a child who is 71 cm tall and weighs 13 kg (Hint: You may want to use the nomogram)

19. Calculate the daily fluid maintenance needs for a child who weighs 13.6 kg. (Hint: Look at Chapter 11)

Comprehensive self-test 4

1. The patient prescription states *doxorubicin HCl (Adriamycin) 80 mg IV once every 21 days*. The patient information leaflet states that the recommended dose for use as a single agent is 60–75 mg/m^2 repeat every 3 weeks. Is this a safe dose for a patient who weighs 39 kg and is 127 cm tall?

2. Prescription: *Clarithromycin oral suspension 7.5 mg/kg PO 12 hourly*. The label reads: 250 mg/5 mL. How many millilitres will you give a child who weighs 18 kg?

3. Prescription: *nitroglycerine 0.6 mg sublingual stat*. The label reads: 0.3 mg tablets. How many tablets will you give the patient?

4. A patient has an IV of 1000 mL Ringer's lactate infusing at 125 mL/h. How many hours will it take to infuse?

5. Calculate the daily fluid maintenance needs for an infant who weighs 2500 g.

6. The prescription indicates *atropine sulphate 0.4 mg IM as a premedication (60 min before theatre)*. The label reads: 1 mg/mL. How many millilitres will you give the patient?

7. Prescription: *octreotide acetate (Sandostatin) 200 mcg subcutaneously q.i.d.* The label reads: 1 mg/mL. How many millilitres will you administer?

8. Prescription: *Labetalol HCl 20 mg IV bolus slowly over 2 min*. The label reads: 5 mg/mL. How many millilitres of this antihypertensive drug will the patient receive per minute?

9. A patient is prescribed *ranitidine (Zantac) 50 mg in 100 mL 5% glucose IV infusion every 8 hours, to be infused over 20 min*. The label reads: 25 mg/mL. Calculate the flow rate in millilitres per minute.

10. Prescription: *Mitomycin-C 20 mg/m^2 IV once every 6 weeks*. Calculate the dose for a patient who has a BSA of 1.62 m^2.

11. Calculate the total daily fluid maintenance for a child who weighs 26 lbs.

12. A child is prescribed *cimetidine (Tagamet) 250 mg IV infusion 6 hourly*. The recommended dose is 5–10 mg/kg every 6 hours. Is this a safe dose for a child who weighs 36 kg?

13. Prescription: *Actrapid insulin 300 units in 150 mL NaCl to infuse at 10 mL/h*. How many units/h is the patient receiving?

14. Prescription: *heparin 5000 units subcutaneous every 12 hours*. The label reads: 10 000 units/mL. How many millilitres will you give the patient?

15. A prescriber orders *vancomycin HCl 500 mg PO every 6 hours* for a child who weighs 50 kg. The pharmacist states that the recommended child's dose is 40 mg/kg/d in three or four divided doses. Is the prescribed dose safe?

Appendices

Appendix A
Answer section

Chapter 1

Diagnostic test of arithmetic

1. $\frac{375}{1000}$ 2. 6.5   3. 3.8   4. 0.025   5. $\frac{18}{7}$

Try these for practice

1. 0.3125   2. 74.4   3. 0.4 and $\frac{2}{5}$ 4. $\frac{1}{3}$ 5. 2

Exercises

1. $0.85 = \dfrac{85 \div 5}{100 \div 5} = \dfrac{17}{20}$ 2. $2.7 = 2\dfrac{7}{10}$ 3. $\dfrac{\overset{5}{\cancel{40}}}{1} \times \dfrac{1}{2} \times \dfrac{9}{\underset{2}{\cancel{16}}} = \dfrac{45}{4} = 11\dfrac{1}{4}$

4. $2\dfrac{3}{5} \div \dfrac{2}{1} = \dfrac{13}{5} \times \dfrac{1}{2} = \dfrac{13}{10} = 1\dfrac{3}{10}$ 5. $\dfrac{15}{1} \div \dfrac{11}{3} = \dfrac{15}{1} \times \dfrac{3}{11} = \dfrac{45}{11} = 4\dfrac{1}{11}$

6. $9.6 \div \dfrac{3}{7} = \dfrac{9.6}{1} \times \dfrac{7}{3} = \dfrac{67.2}{3} = 22.4 = 22\dfrac{2}{5}$ 7. $\dfrac{\overset{14}{\cancel{42}}}{1} \times \dfrac{1}{\underset{3150}{\cancel{9450}}} \times \dfrac{3}{0.02} = \dfrac{42}{63} = \dfrac{2}{3}$

8. $\begin{array}{r} 0.125 \\ 8\overline{)1.000} \\ \underline{8} \\ 20 \\ \underline{16} \\ 40 \\ \underline{40} \\ 0 \end{array} \approx 0.12$ 9. $\begin{array}{r} 0.56 \\ 25\overline{)14.00} \\ \underline{12\,5} \\ 1\,50 \\ \underline{1\,50} \\ 0 \end{array}$ 0.56   10. $5\dfrac{3}{10} = 5.3$ 11. $\begin{array}{r} 0.005 \\ 200\overline{)1.000} \\ \underline{1\,000} \\ 0 \end{array}$ 0.005

12. $\begin{array}{r} 0.013 \\ 75\overline{)1.000} \\ \underline{75} \\ 250 \\ \underline{225} \\ 25 \end{array} \approx 0.01$ 13. $\dfrac{870}{1000} = 8\,7\,0 = 0.87$ 14. $\dfrac{2.73}{100} = 2\,73 = 0.0273$

15. $\begin{array}{r} 2.05 \\ 7\overline{)14.36} \\ \underline{14} \\ 0\,3 \\ \underline{0} \\ 36 \\ \underline{35} \\ 1 \end{array} \approx 2.0$ 16. $0.9\overline{)0.63}$ 0.7 $\begin{array}{r} 0.7 \\ \underline{63} \\ 0 \end{array}$ 17. $0.09\overline{)0.063}$ 0.7 $\begin{array}{r} 0.7 \\ \underline{63} \\ 0 \end{array}$

18. $5\frac{1}{2}\% = 5.5\% = \;\;5.5 = 0.055$

19. $55\% = \;5\,5 = 0.55$

20.
$$\begin{array}{r} 4.\underline{63} \\ \times\,6.21 \\ \hline 4\,63 \\ 92\,6 \\ 2778 \\ \hline 28.\underline{7523} \end{array} \approx 28.75$$

21. $0.\,0\,0\,4 = 0.4$

22. $2.\,3\,4\,5\,6 = 2345.6$

23. $0.03\,\overline{)\,.8\,5\,00}\;\approx 28.3$ with quotient 28.33
$$\begin{array}{r} 6 \\ \hline 2\,5 \\ 2\,4 \\ \hline 1\,0 \\ 9 \\ \hline 10 \\ 9 \\ \hline 1 \end{array}$$

24. $0.1\,2\,\overline{)\,8.5\,0\,000}\;\approx 70.83$ with quotient 70.833
$$\begin{array}{r} 8\,4 \\ \hline 10 \\ 0 \\ \hline 100 \\ 9\,6 \\ \hline 40 \\ 36 \\ \hline 40 \\ 36 \\ \hline 4 \end{array}$$

25. $0.72 \times \dfrac{1}{0.7} = \dfrac{0.72}{70} \Rightarrow .7\,\overline{)\,.7\,20}\;\approx 1.0$ with quotient 1.02
$$\begin{array}{r} 7 \\ \hline 0\,2 \\ 0 \\ \hline 20 \\ 14 \\ \hline 6 \end{array}$$
$$\frac{0.72 \times 100}{0.7 \times 100} = \frac{72}{70} = 1\frac{2}{70}$$
$1\frac{2}{70}$ and 1.0

26. $\dfrac{\frac{2}{3}}{\frac{3}{8}} = 2 \div \dfrac{3}{8} = \dfrac{2}{1} \times \dfrac{8}{3} = \dfrac{16}{3} = 5\frac{1}{3}$

$$\begin{array}{r} 5.33 \\ 3\overline{)16.00} \approx 5.3 \\ 15 \\ \hline 1\,0 \\ 9 \\ \hline 10 \\ 9 \\ \hline 1 \end{array}$$
$5\frac{1}{3}$ and 5.3

27. $\dfrac{\frac{2}{5}}{\frac{500}{100}} \times \dfrac{500}{6} = \dfrac{\frac{2}{5} \times \frac{5}{1}}{6} = \dfrac{2}{6} = \dfrac{1}{3}$

$$\begin{array}{r} .33 \\ 3\overline{)1.00} \approx 0.3 \\ 9 \\ \hline 10 \\ 9 \\ \hline 1 \end{array}$$
$\frac{1}{3}$ and 0.3

28. $\dfrac{26 \times \frac{5}{13}}{\frac{9}{100}} = \dfrac{26}{1} \times \dfrac{5}{13} \div \dfrac{9}{100} = \dfrac{26}{1} \times \dfrac{5}{13} \times \dfrac{100}{9} = \dfrac{1000}{9}$

257

$$9\overline{)1000} \Rightarrow 111\frac{1}{9}$$

$$\begin{array}{r} 111 \\ 9\overline{)1000} \\ \underline{9} \\ 10 \\ \underline{9} \\ 10 \\ \underline{9} \\ 1 \end{array}$$

$$\begin{array}{r} .11 \\ 9\overline{)1.00} \\ \underline{9} \\ 10 \\ \underline{9} \\ 1 \end{array} \quad 111\frac{1}{9} \approx 111.11 \approx 111.1$$

$$111\frac{1}{9} \text{ and } 111.1$$

29. $10.3\% = 1\,0\,.\,3 = 0.103 \approx 0.1$

$0.103 = \dfrac{103}{1000}$

$\frac{103}{1000}$ and 0.1

30. $99.5\% = 9\,9\,.\,5 = 0.995 \approx 1.0$

$0.995 = \dfrac{995 \div 5}{1000 \div 5} = \dfrac{191}{200}$

$\frac{199}{200}$ and 1.0

Chapter 2

Diagnostic questions

1. What is a drug prescription? *A legal document with specific written instructions for the supply of or administration of a licensed named medicine including vaccines to an individually identified person or groups (patient group directive) (NMC 2007).*

2. Who are the main people involved in the prescription process? *The prescriber, the dispenser (or pharmacist), the person administering the drug and the patient.*

3. How many RIGHTS of drug administration are there? *Six: right dose, right time, right route, right patient, right drug, right documentation.*

4. What is the role of a drug package insert also known as Patient Information Leaflet (PiL)? *An information leaflet containing details of the drug chemistry, preparation or side effects.*

5. What does the GENERIC name of a drug mean? *The officially accepted name of a drug (not the brand or proprietary name).*

Try these for practice

1. PO (orally)   2. 28   3. 400 mg   4. lopinavir 80 mg and ritonavir 20 mg

Exercises

1. lopinavir/ritonavir   2. 40 mg per tablet

3. (a) Anusol supp (b) 6 a.m. (c) 3 (d) Ibandronic acid (e) 18 December

4. (a) digoxin, furosemide (b) Metoclopramide (c) 10 mg PO (d) transdermal (e) Cefalexin

5. (a) 5–40 mg in divided doses (b) two weeks
(c) 2 mg/5 mL

6. 9 a.m.   0900 h
   3 p.m.   1500 h
   Noon   1200 h
   6 p.m.   1800 h
   8:15 p.m.   2015 h

2:30 a.m.	0230 h
4:45 p.m.	1645 h
6 a.m.	0600 h
Midnight	0000 h

Chapter 3

Diagnostic questions

1. You are having a tea party with four of your colleagues at work. You have brought a small cake and cut it up equally between the four of you. What is another term for one portion of that cake? *One quarter or 1/4.*

2. One colleague is on a diet and so you eat two portions of the cake. What is another way of communicating this amount? *Two quarters, 2/4 or one half 1/2.*

3. Mr Jones has a fluid restriction. One colleague tells you he has had $^3/_4$ of his allowance and another colleague tells you he has had 75%. Are these different amounts? *Same amounts.*

4. Which is the greater amount, 104 weeks or 2 years? *Both the same – 52 weeks in a year.*

5. A patient must exercise 30 minutes twice a day. He tells you he prefers to exercise 10 minutes six times a day. Will he have enough exercise? *It is the same amount.*

Try these for practice

1. 270 min   2. 115 oz   3. 252 h   4. 6 L/h   5. 1.75 kg/week

Exercises

1. $\dfrac{1.5\ \cancel{min}}{1}\times\dfrac{60\ sec}{1\ \cancel{min}}=90\ sec$ 2. $\dfrac{11\ \cancel{y}}{\underset{1}{\cancel{2}}}\times\dfrac{\overset{6}{\cancel{12}}\ mon}{1\ \cancel{y}}=66\ mon$ 3. $\dfrac{18\ \cancel{d}}{\underset{1}{\cancel{4}}}\times\dfrac{\overset{6}{\cancel{24}}\ h}{1\ \cancel{d}}=108\ h$

4. $\dfrac{3\ \cancel{h}}{\underset{1}{\cancel{4}}}\times\dfrac{\overset{15}{\cancel{60}}\ min}{1\ \cancel{h}}=45\ min$ 5. $\dfrac{\overset{17}{\cancel{51}}\ \cancel{mon}}{1}\times\dfrac{1\ y}{\underset{4}{\cancel{12}}\ \cancel{mon}}=\dfrac{17\ y}{4}=4\dfrac{1}{4}\,y$

6. 3 L × 1000 mL/1 L = 3000 mL   7. 3 kg × 1000 gm/1 kg = 3000 gm

8. 100 cm/sec × 1 m/100 cm = 1 m/sec

9. 30 L/min × 1 min/60 sec = 0.5 L/sec

10. 60 km/hour × 1000 m/km × 1 h/60 min = 1000 m/min

11. $2700\ \cancel{sec}\times\dfrac{\cancel{min}}{60\ \cancel{sec}}\times\dfrac{h}{60\ \cancel{min}}=\dfrac{27\ h}{36}=\dfrac{3}{4}\,h$ 12. $\overset{240}{\cancel{1680}}\ \cancel{h}\times\dfrac{\cancel{day}}{24\ \cancel{h}}\times\dfrac{week}{\underset{1}{\cancel{7}\ \cancel{days}}}=10\ week$

13. $\dfrac{1\ 209\ 600\ \cancel{sec}}{1}\times\dfrac{1\ \cancel{min}}{60\ \cancel{sec}}\times\dfrac{1\ \cancel{h}}{60\ \cancel{min}}\times\dfrac{1\ \cancel{day}}{24\ \cancel{h}}\times\dfrac{1\ week}{7\ \cancel{days}}=2\ week$

14. $\dfrac{5\ \cancel{cases}}{1}\times\dfrac{24\ \cancel{cans}}{\cancel{case}}\times\dfrac{330\ \cancel{mL}}{\cancel{can}}\times\dfrac{10\ \cancel{g}}{100\ \cancel{mL}}\times\dfrac{1\ kg}{1000\ \cancel{g}}=3.96\ kg$

Chapter 4

Diagnostic questions

1. Which is larger 5.17 or 5.38? *5.38*

2. Which is smaller 2.19 or 2.64? *2.19*

3. Put these in size order, the largest first:
   75.1, 25.7, 25.762, 0.34, 3.44 *Answer: 75.1, 25.762, 25.7, 3.44, 0.34*

4. Put these in order, the smallest first:
   0.96, 0.547, 0.009, 1.76, 0.19 *Answer: 0.009, 0.19, 0.547, 0.96, 1.76*

5. Write three and four tenths as a decimal using digits. *Answer: 3.4*

Try these for practice

1. (a) 1000 mL (b) 10000 mL (c) 1000 g (d) 1000 mg (e) 1000 mcg (f) 10000 mcg

2. 0.01 g   3. 5000 mcg   4. 1.8 L   5. 1500 mL

Exercises

1. $\dfrac{400\ \text{mg}}{1} \times \dfrac{1\ \text{g}}{1000\ \text{mg}} = \dfrac{4}{10}\ \text{g} = 0.4\ \text{g}$ 2. $\dfrac{0.003\ \text{g}}{1} \times \dfrac{1000\ \text{mg}}{1\ \text{g}} = 3\ \text{mg}$

3. $\dfrac{0.07\ \text{g}}{1} \times \dfrac{1000\ \text{mg}}{1\ \text{g}} = 70\ \text{mg}$ 4. $\dfrac{3\ \text{L}}{1} \times \dfrac{1000\ \text{mL}}{1\ \text{L}} = 3000\ \text{mL}$

5. $\dfrac{2500\ \text{mL}}{1} \times \dfrac{1\ \text{L}}{1000\ \text{mL}} = \dfrac{25}{20}\ \text{L} = 2.5\ \text{L}$ 6. $\dfrac{600\ \text{mcg}}{1} \times \dfrac{1\ \text{mg}}{1000\ \text{mcg}} = \dfrac{6}{10}\ \text{mg} = 0.6\ \text{mg}$

7. $\dfrac{40\ \text{mg}}{1} \times \dfrac{1000\ \text{mcg}}{1\ \text{mg}} = 40\,000\ \text{mcg}$ 8. $\dfrac{520\ \text{mcg}}{1} \times \dfrac{1\ \text{mg}}{1000\ \text{mcg}} = \dfrac{52}{100}\ \text{mg} = 0.52\ \text{mg}$

9. $\dfrac{50\ \text{mg}}{1} \times \dfrac{1\ \text{g}}{1000\ \text{mg}} = \dfrac{5}{100}\ \text{g} = 0.05\ \text{g}$ 10. 8 h/1 × L/2 h × 1000 mL/1 L = 2000 mL

11. $\dfrac{3400\ \text{g}}{1} \times \dfrac{1\ \text{kg}}{1000\ \text{g}} = \dfrac{34}{10}\ \text{kg} = 3.4\ \text{kg}$

12. First convert ft to in: 5 ft × 12 in/1 ft = 60 in
    Then add 2 in: 60 in + 2 in = 62 in
    Then convert in to cm: 62 in × 2.54 cm = 157.48 cm

13. 165 lbs × 453.59 g/1 × 1 kg/1000 g = 74.84 kg

Chapter 5

Diagnostic questions

1. You wish to give your patient 1 g of paracetamol. The container indicates each tablet is 500 mg. How many tablets do you give? *Answer: 2 tablets.*

2. The drug Atropine 600 mcg is to be given. How many milligrams is this? *Answer: 0.6 mg.*

3. Codeine 0.08 g is prescribed to a patient. How many milligrams is this? *Answer: 80 mg.*

4. A patient is to have 0.125 mg digoxin. You have a stock of digoxin 0.0625 mg. How many tablets do you give? *Answer: 2 tablets.*

5. A patient is to drink one and half litres of fluid over 24 hours. How many mLs is that? *Answer: 1500 mL.*

Case study 5.1

1. 650 mL + 150 mL + 200 mL = 1000 mL   1500 mL − 1000 mL = 500 mL

2. (a) $\dfrac{375 \text{ mL}}{1} \times \dfrac{390 \text{ mg}}{250 \text{ mL}} \times \dfrac{g}{1000 \text{ mg}} = \dfrac{585}{1000 \text{ g}} = 0.585 \text{ g}$ (b) 2 g − 0.59 g = 1.41 g

3. (a) $\overset{4}{80 \text{ mg}} \times \dfrac{1 \text{ tab}}{\underset{1}{20 \text{ mg}}} = 4$ tab (for stat dose)   (b) $\overset{3}{60 \text{ mg}} \times \dfrac{1 \text{ tab}}{\underset{1}{20 \text{ mg}}} = 3$ tab (12 h later)

   4 tab + 3 tab = 7 tab within first 20 hours

4. $5 \text{ days} \times \dfrac{24 \text{ mmol}}{\text{day}} = 120 \text{ mmol}$

5. (a) t.i.d. means 3 times per day   (b) $\dfrac{2 \text{ days}}{1} \times \dfrac{3 \text{ doses}}{\text{day}} \times \dfrac{\overset{5}{100 \text{ mg}}}{\text{dose}} \times \dfrac{5 \text{ mL}}{\underset{1}{20 \text{ mg}}} = 150 \text{ mL}$

6. $3 \text{ mg} \times \dfrac{\text{tab}}{1 \text{ mg}} = 3$ tab

7. $0.25 \text{ mg} \times \dfrac{1000 \text{ mcg}}{1 \text{ mg}} = 250 \text{ mcg}$ one 200 mcg tab and one 50 mcg tab.

8. $7 \text{ days} \times \dfrac{125 \text{ mg}}{\text{day}} = 875 \text{ mg}$

Practice reading labels

1. $0.05 \text{ g} \times \dfrac{1000 \text{ mg}}{g} \times \dfrac{\text{tab}}{50 \text{ mg}} = \dfrac{50}{50} \text{ tab} = 1$ tab   2. $200 \text{ mg} \times \dfrac{\text{tab}}{100 \text{ mg}} = 2$ tab

3. $0.12 \text{ g} \times \dfrac{1000 \text{ mg}}{g} = \overset{2}{120 \text{ mg}} \times \dfrac{\text{cap}}{\underset{1}{60 \text{ mg}}} = 2$ cap   4. $\overset{2}{40 \text{ mg}} \times \dfrac{5 \text{ mL}}{\underset{1}{20 \text{ mg}}} = 10$ mL

5. $0.25 \text{ g} \times \dfrac{1000 \text{ mg}}{g} = 250 \text{ mg} \times \dfrac{\text{tab}}{250 \text{ mg}} = 1$ tab   6. $\overset{2}{800 \text{ mg}} \times \dfrac{\text{tab}}{\underset{1}{400 \text{ mg}}} = 2$ tab

7. $\overset{2}{10 \text{ mg}} \times \dfrac{\text{tab}}{\underset{1}{5 \text{ mg}}} = 2$ tab   8. $0.6 \text{ g} \times \dfrac{1000 \text{ mg}}{g} \times \dfrac{\text{tab}}{300 \text{ mg}} = \dfrac{600}{300} \text{ tab} = 2$ tab

9. $\overset{1}{100 \text{ mg}} \times \dfrac{10 \text{ mL}}{\underset{1}{100 \text{ mg}}} = 10$ mL   10. $\overset{1}{125 \text{ mcg}} \times \dfrac{2 \text{ mL}}{\underset{4}{500 \text{ mcg}}} = \dfrac{1}{2} \text{ mL} = 0.5$ mL

11. $0.4\ \text{g} \times \dfrac{1000\ \text{mg}}{\text{g}} \times \dfrac{\text{tab}}{200\ \text{mg}} = \dfrac{4}{2}\ \text{tab} = 2\ \text{tab}$ 12. $5\ \text{mg} \times \dfrac{\text{tab}}{2.5\ \text{mg}} = \dfrac{5}{2.5}\ \text{tab} = 2\ \text{tab}$

13. $\overset{4}{80}\ \text{mg} \times \dfrac{\text{cap}}{\underset{1}{20}\ \text{mg}} = 4\ \text{cap}$ 14. $0.05\ \text{mg} \times \dfrac{5\ \text{mL}}{5\ \text{mg}} = 0.05\ \text{mL}$

15. $10\ \text{mg} \times \dfrac{1\ \text{cap}}{10\ \text{mg}} = 1\ \text{cap}$ 16. $0.1\ \text{mg} \times \dfrac{1000\ \text{mcg}}{\text{mg}} \times \dfrac{1\ \text{mL}}{100\ \text{mcg}} = 1\ \text{mL}$

17. $0.08\ \text{g} \times \dfrac{1000\ \text{mg}}{\text{g}} \times \dfrac{\text{tab}}{40\ \text{mg}} = \dfrac{8}{4}\ \text{tab} = 2\ \text{tab}$ 18. $130\ \text{mg} \times \dfrac{\text{mL}}{80\ \text{mg}} = \dfrac{13}{8}\ \text{mL} \approx 1.6\ \text{mL}$

19. $\overset{3}{75}\ \text{mg} \times \dfrac{\text{cap}}{\underset{1}{25}\ \text{mg}} = 3\ \text{cap}$ 20. $\overset{2}{8}\ \text{mg} \times \dfrac{\text{tab}}{\underset{1}{4}\ \text{mg}} = 2\ \text{tab}$

Try these for practice

1. (a) 2 tablets (b) 0.08 g   2. using nomogram BSA = 1.67 = 83.5 mg; using Mosteller calculation BSA = 1.70 = 85 mg   3. 6 capsules   4. One 50 mg and 2 15 mg tablets

Exercises

1. $40\ \text{mg} \times \dfrac{\text{g}}{1000\ \text{mg}} \times \dfrac{\text{tab}}{0.02\ \text{g}} = \dfrac{4}{2}\ \text{tab} = 2\ \text{tab}$

2. $500\ \text{mcg} \times \dfrac{\text{mg}}{1000\ \text{mcg}} \times \dfrac{\text{mL}}{0.05\ \text{mg}} = \dfrac{50}{5}\ \text{mL} = 10\ \text{mL}$

3. $\overset{3}{75}\ \text{mg} \times \dfrac{\text{tab}}{\underset{1}{25}\ \text{mg}} = 3\ \text{tab per dose} \times 3\ \text{doses per day} = 9\ \text{tab}$

4. $7\ \text{days} \times \dfrac{200\ \text{mg}}{\text{day}} \times \dfrac{\text{tab}}{200\ \text{mg}} = 7\ \text{tab}$

5. $40\ \text{kg} \times \dfrac{50\ \text{mg}}{\text{kg}} \times \dfrac{\text{tab}}{500\ \text{mg}} = \dfrac{20}{5} = 4\ \text{tab daily which is 2 tab per dose}$

6. $0.015\ \text{g} \times \dfrac{1000\ \text{mg}}{\text{g}} \times \dfrac{\text{tab}}{7.5\ \text{mg}} = \dfrac{15}{7.5}\ \text{tab} = 2\ \text{tab}$

7. $\dfrac{\overset{6}{150}\ \text{mg}}{\text{day}} \times \dfrac{\text{tab}}{\underset{1}{25}\ \text{mg}} = \dfrac{6\ \text{tab}}{\text{day}}\ \text{in 3 divided doses means give 2 tablets per dose}$

8. $\overset{3}{75}\ \text{mg} \times \dfrac{\text{cap}}{\underset{1}{25}\ \text{mg}} = 3\ \text{cap}$

9. Patient receives warfarin on Mon., Wed., Fri. and Sun.

$$\dfrac{6.5\ \text{mg}}{\text{dose}} \times \dfrac{4\ \text{dose}}{\text{wk}} = 26\ \text{mg per week}$$

10. 500 mg on day 1 and 250 mg on next 4 days means
    500 mg + 1000 mg = 1500 mg in total

Chapter 6

Diagnostic questions

1. List three types of injection routes. *Answer: subcutaneous, intramuscular, intravenous, intrademal, etc.*

2. A patient is to have 25 units of insulin. The stock insulin is 100 units per mL. Do you draw up the insulin in any syringe as mLs or do you use a specific syringe? *Answer: Use an insulin syringe for accurate calibrations to measure the insulin.*

3. A patient is being prepared for surgery and due to have an injection of Atropine 600 mcg. You need to draw up 0.6 mL. What is the best syringe to use: 1 mL, 2 mL, 5 mL, 10 mL? *Answer: 1 mL for more accuracy or 2 mL if not available – use the smallest possible for accuracy.*

4. If a patient is prescribed 2 types of insulin can they be drawn up in the same syringe? *Answer: Depends on the type of insulin – it is possible if they are compatible. See the section on insulin.*

5. In what way can syringes cause drug errors? *Answer: using the wrong size syringe and inaccurate determination of dose, wrong route or technique, drawing up too many syringes and not labelling them.*

Case study 6.1

1. (a) $75 \text{ mg} \times \dfrac{\text{mL}}{100 \text{ mg}} = \dfrac{75}{100} \text{ mL} = 0.75 \text{ mL}$

   (b) the 1 mL syringe

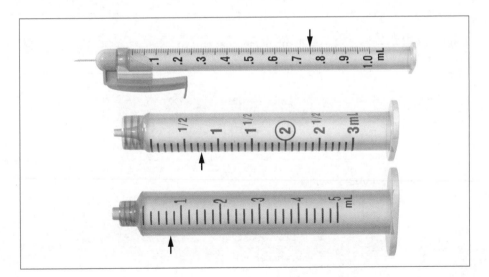

2. (a) $25 \text{ mg} \times \dfrac{\text{mL}}{25 \text{ mg}} = 1 \text{ mL of promethazine}$

(b)

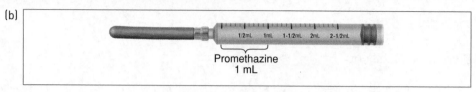

Promethazine
1 mL

3.

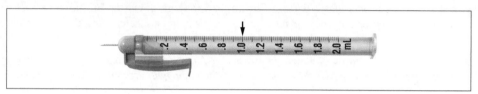

9 mL

4. $12.5 \, \cancel{mg} \times \dfrac{mL}{12.5 \, \cancel{mg}} = \dfrac{12.5}{12.5} \, mL = 1.0 \, mL$

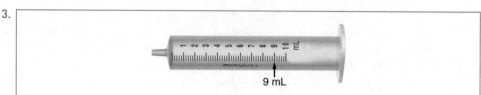

5. (a) $75 \, \cancel{mg} \times \dfrac{mL}{100 \, \cancel{mg}} = \dfrac{75}{100} \, mL = 0.75 \, mL \text{ pethidine}$

(b)

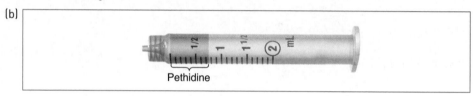

Pethidine

6. (a) $1 \, \cancel{g} \times \dfrac{\overset{20}{\cancel{1000}} \, \cancel{mg}}{1 \, \cancel{g}} \times \dfrac{mL}{\underset{1}{\cancel{50} \, \cancel{mg}}} = 20 \, mL \text{ of Meropenem}$

(b)

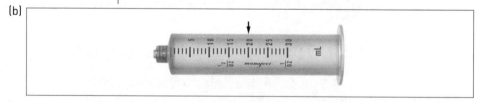

7. (a) 13 units + 6 units = 19 units

(b)

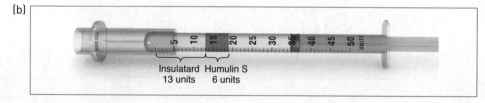

Insulatard   Humulin S
13 units   6 units

(c) To avoid contamination of individual vials of insulin. Other benefits could be ease of
storage and reduction of errors in drawing up.

Try these for practice

1. 1 mL tuberculin syringe; 0.72 mL

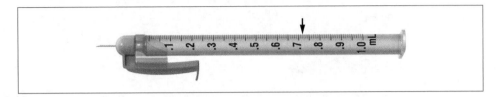

2. 12 mL syringe; 6.8 mL

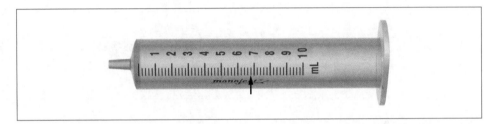

3. 3 mL syringe; 2.8 mL

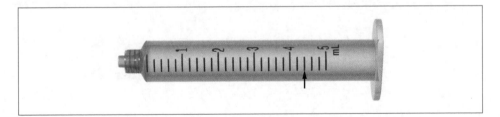

4. 5 mL syringe; 4.4 mL

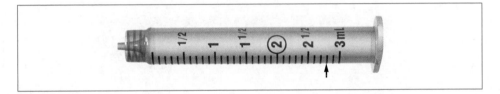

5. (a) 100 unit insulin syringe

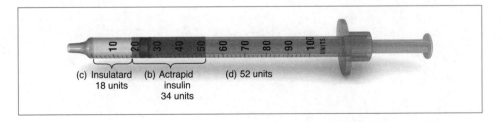

265

Exercises

1. 1 mL tuberculin syringe; 0.62 mL

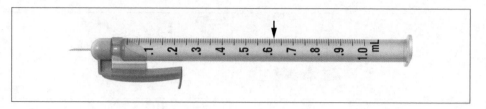

2. 50 unit Lo-Dose insulin syringe; 28 units

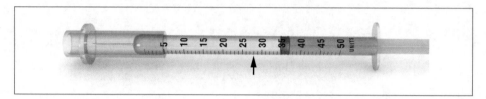

3. 5 mL syringe; 3.6 mL

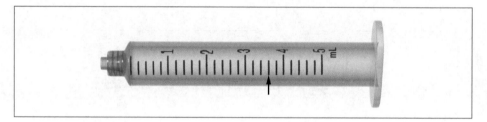

4. 3 mL syringe; 1.4 mL

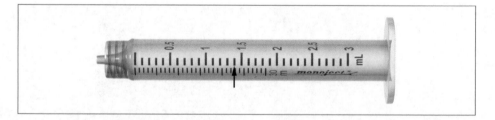

5. 30 mL syringe; 13 mL

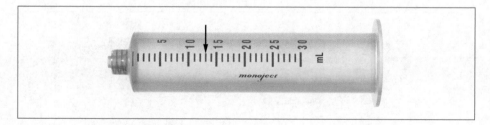

6. 12 mL syringe; 9.6 mL

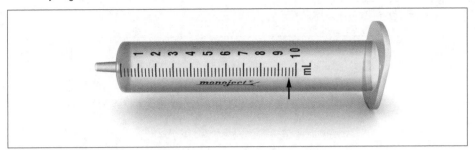

7. 50 unit Lo-Dose insulin syringe; 32 units

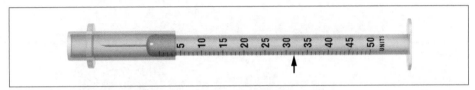

8. 100 unit insulin syringe; 56 units

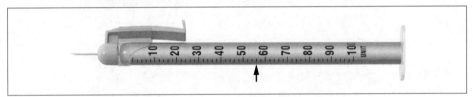

9. 1 mL tuberculin syringe; 0.37 mL

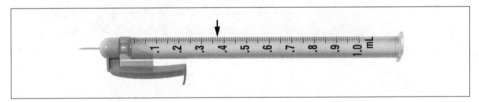

10. 100 unit insulin syringe; 51 units

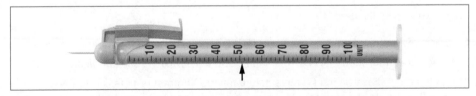

11.

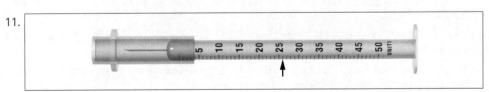

12. $600 \text{ mg} \times \dfrac{1 \text{ mL}}{400 \text{ mg}} = 1.5 \text{ mL}$

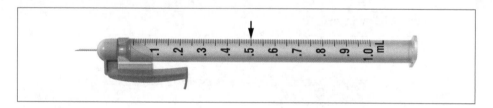

13. $200 \text{ mg} \times \dfrac{5 \text{ mL}}{250 \text{ mg}} = 4 \text{ mL}$

14. $0.2 \text{ mg} \times \dfrac{\text{mL}}{0.4 \text{ mg}} = \dfrac{0.2}{0.4} \text{ mL} = 0.5 \text{ mL}$

Chapter 7

Diagnostic questions

1. How many grams of glucose are there in 100 mL of a 5% glucose solution? *Answer: 5 g.*

2. What is the other name for 'normal saline' solution? *Answer: Sodium Chloride 0.9%.*

3. A patient is to have an intravenous solution with 20 mmol of potassium. Does millimoles (mmol) refers to the weight, colour or type of potassium used in the solution? *Answer: Weight.*

4. A 1 in 1000 solution is stronger (more concentrated) than a 1 in 100 solution. True or False? *Answer: False it is weaker.*

5. Drugs can be measured as 'units' as well as traditional weights like grams and milligrams. True or False? *Answer: True: Examples include heparin and insulin.*

Case study 7.1

1. 0.5 mL – use 1 mL syringe

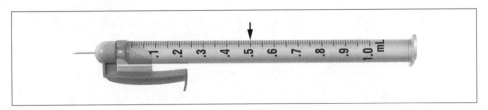

2. 180 mg = 120 mg + 60 mg

   Use one 120 mg and one 60 mg tablet for each dose. Administer the two tablets daily.

3. $\overset{1}{\cancel{20}} \ \cancel{\text{mmol}} \times \dfrac{15 \text{ mL}}{\underset{2}{\cancel{40} \ \cancel{\text{mmol}}}} = 7.5 \text{ mL}$

4. Administer one 75 mg tablet.

5. $\overset{2}{\cancel{1000}} \ \cancel{\text{mg}} \times \dfrac{\text{tab}}{\underset{1}{\cancel{500} \ \cancel{\text{mg}}}} = 2 \text{ tab}$

6. Withdraw 10 units of Humulin S insulin, then into the same syringe withdraw 38 units of Humulin I insulin for a total of 48 units.

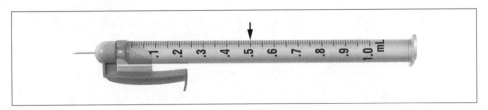

7. $1 \ \cancel{\text{L}} \times \dfrac{1000 \ \cancel{\text{mL}}}{1 \ \cancel{\text{L}}} \times \dfrac{0.9 \text{ g (NaCl)}}{100 \ \cancel{\text{mL}}} = 9 \text{ g}$

Try these for practice

1. $\dfrac{\text{Drug}}{\text{Solution}} = \dfrac{\overset{1}{\cancel{80}} \ \cancel{\text{mg}}}{\underset{4}{\cancel{320} \text{ mL}}} \times \dfrac{1 \text{ g}}{1000 \ \cancel{\text{mg}}} = \dfrac{1 \text{ g}}{4000 \text{ mL}} \qquad \dfrac{1}{4000} = 0.00025 = 0.025\%$

2. $1 \ \cancel{\text{L}} \times \dfrac{1000 \ \cancel{\text{mL}}}{1 \ \cancel{\text{L}}} \times \dfrac{10 \ \cancel{\text{g}}}{100 \ \cancel{\text{mL}}} \times \dfrac{1 \text{ tab}}{5 \ \cancel{\text{g}}} = 20 \text{ tab}$

   Take 20 tablets and dissolve with water, then add more water to the level of 1 L.

3. $20 \ \cancel{\text{g}} \times \dfrac{\overset{4}{\cancel{100} \text{ mL}}}{\underset{1}{\cancel{25} \ \cancel{\text{g}}}} = 80 \text{ mL}$

4. $$\dfrac{200\ mL \times \dfrac{5\ g}{100\ mL}}{\dfrac{20\ g}{100\ mL}} = \text{Amount of stock}$$

$$\cancel{200}^{10}\ mL \times \dfrac{5\ \cancel{g}}{\cancel{100\ mL}} \times \dfrac{\cancel{100\ mL}}{\cancel{20\ g}_1} = 50\ mL$$

Take 50 mL of the stock solution and add water to the level of 200 mL.

5. $\left(\dfrac{0.5\ mg}{2\ mL}\right) \times \dfrac{1000\ mcg}{1\ mg} = \left(\dfrac{500\ mcg}{2\ mL}\right)$

Exercises

1. $\dfrac{Drug}{Solution} = \dfrac{\cancel{15}^{1}\ mL}{\cancel{750}_{50}\ mL} = \dfrac{1}{50} = \dfrac{2}{100}$

The strength is 1:50 or 2%

2. $\dfrac{Drug}{Solution} = \dfrac{\cancel{60}\ g}{\cancel{2}\ \cancel{L}} \times \dfrac{1\ \cancel{L}}{\cancel{100}\ mL} = \dfrac{3\ g}{100\ mL}$

The strength is 3:100 or 3%

3. $\cancel{300}\ \cancel{mL} \times \dfrac{0.9\ g}{\cancel{100\ mL}} = 2.7\ g$

4. $120\ \cancel{mL} \times \dfrac{\cancel{25}^{5}\ mg}{\cancel{5\ mL}_1} = 600\ mg$

5. $20\ \cancel{mg} \times \dfrac{\cancel{5}^{1}\ mL}{\cancel{25}_{5}\ mg} = 4\ mL$

6. $\cancel{18}^{3}\ \cancel{g} \times \dfrac{100\ mL}{\cancel{6}_1\ \cancel{g}} = 300\ mL$

7. $\cancel{300}\ \cancel{mg} \times \dfrac{\cancel{g}}{\cancel{1000}\ \cancel{mg}} \times \dfrac{\cancel{100}\ mL}{4\ \cancel{g}} = \dfrac{30}{4}\ mL = 7.5\ mL$

8. $\dfrac{Drug}{Solution} = \dfrac{\cancel{120}\ mL}{\cancel{600}\ mL} = \dfrac{1}{5},\ 1:5\ or\ 20\%$

9. $\dfrac{Drug}{Solution} = \dfrac{\cancel{2000}^{2}\ mg}{1\ \cancel{L}} \times \dfrac{1\ \cancel{L}}{\cancel{1000}_1\ mL} \times \dfrac{1\ g}{1000\ \cancel{mg}} = \dfrac{2\ g}{1000\ mL}$

$\dfrac{2}{1000} = \dfrac{1}{500},\ 1:500\ or\ 0.2\%$

10. $35\ \cancel{mg} \times \dfrac{5\ mL}{\cancel{5\ mg}} = 35\ mL$

11. $\dfrac{\cancel{10}\ \cancel{mg}}{mL} \times \dfrac{g}{\cancel{1000}\ \cancel{mg}} = \dfrac{1\ g}{100\ mL}$

$\dfrac{1}{100} = 1\%$

12. $12\ \cancel{mL} \times \dfrac{\cancel{5}^{1}\ mg}{\cancel{5}_1\ \cancel{mL}} = 12\ mg$

Chapter 8

Diagnostic questions

1. A medication which is stated on the package as 10 mg/10 mL is the same as 1 mg/mL. True or False? *Answer: True.*

2. You need to prepare 375 mcg of a drug and it is available as 500 mcg in 5 mL. On estimation, before calculation, do you need more or less than 3 mL? *Answer: More than 3 mL (equals 100 mcg per mL).*

3. To reconstitute a powder drug, the liquid you add (the diluent) is always water for injection. True or False? *Answer: False. Sometimes it may be sodium chloride 0.9%. This is indicated on the summary of product characteristics (SPC) leaflet.*

4. After reconstituting a drug there may be an additional volume, e.g. adding 2.5 mL of diluent may lead to a total final volume of 3 mL. Why is this? *Answer: Due to the volume added by the powdered drug.*

5. A cluttered and untidy clinical preparation room is one factor in drug errors. Fact or Fiction? *Answer: Fact.*

Case study 8.1

1. (a) $2 \text{ mg} \times \dfrac{\text{mL}}{5 \text{ mg}} = \dfrac{2}{5} \text{ mL} = 0.4 \text{ mL}$ (b) 2 mg/mL = 72p 2×1 mg/mL = £1.44

5 mg/mL ampoule = £1.30. Thus it would be cheaper to use one 5 mg/mL ampoule. Caution needed when discarding the remainder of the drug – ensure it is according to local policy.

2. (a) $5000 \text{ units} \times \dfrac{\text{mL}}{20\,000 \text{ units}} = 0.25 \text{ mL}$

(b) 5000 units/mL, therefore 1 mL ampoule contains 1×5000 units.

Thus: 5000 units/5000 units $\times 1 = 1$ mL = 54p (one whole ampoule)

5000 units/mL, therefore 5 mL ampoule contains 5×5000 units = 25 000 units

Thus: 5000 units/25 000 units $\times 5 = 1$ mL from a 5 mL ampoule at 74p.

The most cost effective is 5000 units in 1 mL ampoule (54p).

3. $5 \text{ mg} \times \dfrac{\text{mL}}{1 \text{ mg}} = 5 \text{ mL}$ 4. $68 \text{ kg} \times \dfrac{7.5 \text{ mg}}{\text{kg}} = 510 \text{ mg}$

5. $\dfrac{30 \text{ mg}}{\text{dose}} \times \dfrac{\text{mL}}{30 \text{ mg}} \times \dfrac{4 \text{ dose}}{\text{day}} = 4 \text{ mL in 24 hours}$

6. $\dfrac{400 \text{ mg}}{\text{day}} \times \dfrac{250 \text{ mL}}{400 \text{ mg}} \times 5 \text{ days} = 1250 \text{ mL}$ 7. $0.5 \text{ mg} \times \dfrac{\text{cap}}{0.5 \text{ mg}} = 1 \text{ cap}$

8. $10 \text{ mg} \times \dfrac{\text{tab}}{5 \text{ mg}} = 2 \text{ tab}$ 9. (a) 5 mg (b) 1 tab   10. $20 \text{ mg} \times \dfrac{\text{tab}}{10 \text{ mg}} = 2 \text{ tab}$

Try these for practice

1. (a) $\overset{3}{750}\ \text{mg} \times \dfrac{1\ \text{g}}{\underset{4}{1000}\ \text{mg}} \times \dfrac{3\ \text{mL}}{1\ \text{g}} = \dfrac{9}{4}\ \text{mL} = 2.25\ \text{mL} \approx 2.3\ \text{mL}$ (b) 5 mL syringe

2. (a) $75\ \text{mg} \times \dfrac{2\ \text{mL}}{100\ \text{mg}} = \dfrac{6}{4}\ \text{mL} = 1.5\ \text{mL}$ (b) 5 mL syringe

   Change 3 (b) to 5 mL syringe

3. (a) $61\ \text{kg} \times 0.05/\text{kg} = 3.05\ \text{mg}$ (rounded up to 3.1 mg) (b) $3.1\ \text{mg} \times \dfrac{2\ \text{mL}}{2\ \text{mg}} = 3.1\ \text{mL}$

4. (a) $8000\ \text{units} \times \dfrac{\text{mL}}{10\,000\ \text{units}} = 0.8\ \text{mL}$ 5. (a) $1\ \text{g} \times \dfrac{\text{tab}}{0.5\ \text{g}} = 2\ \text{tab}$

   (b) $2\ \text{g} \times \dfrac{2.5\ \text{mL}}{1\ \text{g}} = 5\ \text{mL}$

Exercises

1. $750\ \text{mg} \times \dfrac{\text{mL}}{250\ \text{mg}} = 3\ \text{mL}$

2. (a) $70\ \text{kg} \times \dfrac{0.49\ \text{mcg}}{\text{kg}} \times \dfrac{1\ \text{mL}}{40\ \text{mcg}} = 0.857\ \text{mL}$ (rounded up to 0.86 mL) (b) 1 mL syringe

3. (a) $1200\ \text{mg} \times \dfrac{1\ \text{g}}{1000\ \text{mg}} = 1.2\ \text{g}$ (use the 2 g vial) (b) $1200\ \text{mg} \times \dfrac{\text{mL}}{330\ \text{mg}} = 3.6\ \text{mL}$

4. $\overset{1}{500}\ \text{mg} \times \dfrac{1\ \text{g}}{\underset{2}{1000}\ \text{mg}} \times \dfrac{2.5\ \text{mL}}{1\ \text{g}} = 1.25\ \text{mL} \approx 1.3\ \text{mL}$ 5. $\overset{2}{50}\ \text{mg} \times \dfrac{\text{vial}}{\underset{1}{25}\ \text{mg}} = 2\ \text{vials}$

6. (a) $6000\ \text{units} \times \dfrac{\text{mL}}{20\,000\ \text{units}} = 0.3\ \text{mL}$ (b) 1 mL syringe   7. $60\ \text{mg} \times \dfrac{\text{mL}}{40\ \text{mg}} = 1.5\ \text{mL}$

8. (a) $5\ \text{mg} \times \dfrac{\text{mL}}{15\ \text{mg}} = 0.33\ \text{mL}$ (b) 1 mL syringe   9. $30\ \text{mg} \times \dfrac{\text{mL}}{40\ \text{mg}} = 0.75\ \text{mL}$

10. $3\ \text{mg} \times \dfrac{\text{mL}}{4\ \text{mg}} = 0.75\ \text{mL}$

11. 17 mmol/L (320 mg/dL) is between 15.1 and 19 mmol/L (281–340 md/dL) so give 6 units

12. (a) $3500\ \text{units} \times \dfrac{\text{mL}}{5000\ \text{units}} = 0.7\ \text{mL}$ (b) 1 mL syringe

13. (a) $0.2\ \text{mg} \times \dfrac{\text{mL}}{0.4\ \text{mg}} = 0.5\ \text{mL}$ (b) 1 mL syringe

14. $12.5\ \text{mg} \times \dfrac{\text{mL}}{50\ \text{mg}} = 0.25\ \text{mL}$ 15. $\overset{8}{40}\ \text{mg} \times \dfrac{\text{mL}}{\underset{5}{25}\ \text{mg}} = 1.6\ \text{mL}$

Chapter 9

Diagnostic questions

1. The rate at which fluids are administered to a patient is in a volume over time (mLs per hour or Litres per hour). True or False? *Answer: True.*

2. Convert 1.5 L of fluid over 6 hours to mLs per hour. *Answer: 250 mL per hour.*

3. Convert 300 mL per hour to mLs per minute. *Answer: 5 mL per minute.*

4. If 1 mL of fluid contains 10 drops, how many drops are there in 50 mL? *Answer: 500 drops.*

5. Flow rate of fluids is in drops per minute. Identify two methods by which this is controlled in clinical settings? *Answer: electronic pumps or roller clamps on giving sets.*

Case study 9.1

1. $\dfrac{1000 \text{ mL}}{8 \text{ h}} = 125 \text{ mL/h}$ 2. $\dfrac{125 \text{ mL}}{\text{h}} \times \dfrac{1 \text{ h}}{60 \text{ min}} \times \dfrac{15 \text{ drops}}{\text{mL}} = 31 \text{ drops/min}$

3. $\begin{array}{l} 1900 \\ +0800 \\ \hline 2700 \end{array}$ $\begin{array}{l} 2700 \\ -2400 \\ \hline 0300 \end{array}$ 0300 hours

4. $1000 \text{ mL} \times \dfrac{5 \text{ g}}{100 \text{ mL}} = 50 \text{ g glucose}$

$1000 \text{ mL} \times \dfrac{0.45 \text{ g}}{100 \text{ mL}} = 4.5 \text{ g NaCl}$

5. $\dfrac{100 \text{ mL}}{60 \text{ min}} \times \dfrac{60 \text{ min}}{\text{h}} = \dfrac{100 \text{ mL}}{\text{h}}$

6. (a) $800 \text{ mL} \times \dfrac{3 \text{ mL}}{4 \text{ mL}} = 600 \text{ mL needed}$

$600 \text{ mL} \times \dfrac{\text{mL}}{30 \text{ mL}} \times \dfrac{\text{can}}{250 \text{ mL}} = 2 \text{ cans}$

(b) $\dfrac{800 \text{ mL}}{7 \text{ h}} = 114 \text{ mL/h}$

7. $0.5 \text{ mg} \times \dfrac{1 \text{ mL}}{1 \text{ mg}} = 0.5 \text{ mL}$ 8. $200 \text{ mg} \times \dfrac{\text{mL}}{10 \text{ mg}} = 20 \text{ mL}$ 9. $100 \text{ mg} \times \dfrac{\overset{1}{15} \text{ mL}}{\underset{4}{60} \text{ mg}} = 25 \text{ mL}$

Try these for practice

1. $\dfrac{500 \text{ mL}}{8 \text{ h}} \times \dfrac{1 \text{ h}}{60 \text{ min}} \times \dfrac{10 \text{ drops}}{\text{mL}} = 10 \text{ drops/min}$

2. $\dfrac{575 \text{ mL}}{4 \text{ h}} \times \dfrac{1 \text{ h}}{\underset{4}{60} \text{ min}} \times \dfrac{\overset{1}{15} \text{ drops}}{\text{mL}} = 36 \text{ drops/min}$ 3. $\dfrac{500 \text{ mL}}{4 \text{ h}} = 125 \text{ mL/h}$

4. $\dfrac{27 \text{ drops}}{\text{min}} \times \dfrac{\text{mL}}{15 \text{ drops}} \times \dfrac{\overset{4}{60 \text{ min}}}{h} = 108 \text{ mL/h}$ 5. $\dfrac{400 \text{ mL}}{6 \text{ h}} = 67 \text{ mL/h}$

Exercises

1. $\dfrac{750 \text{ mL}}{8 \text{ h}} \times \dfrac{1 \text{ h}}{60 \text{ min}} \times \dfrac{10 \text{ drops}}{\text{mL}} = 16 \text{ drops/min}$ 2. $\dfrac{375 \text{ mL}}{3 \text{ h}} = 125 \text{ mL/h}$

3. $\dfrac{50 \text{ mL}}{h} \times \dfrac{1 \text{ h}}{60 \text{ min}} \times \dfrac{10 \text{ drops}}{\text{mL}} = 8 \text{ drops/min}$ 4. $1000 \text{ mL} \times \dfrac{h}{125 \text{ mL}} = 8 \text{ h}$

5. $\dfrac{500 \text{ mL}}{3 \text{ h}} = 167 \text{ mL/h} = 167 \text{ mcdrop/min}$

6. (a) $\dfrac{1500 \text{ mL}}{12 \text{ h}} \times \dfrac{1 \text{ h}}{\underset{3}{60 \text{ min}}} \times \dfrac{\overset{1}{20 \text{ drop}}}{\text{mL}} = 42 \text{ drops/min}$

   (b) $\dfrac{1200 \text{ mL}}{9 \text{ h}} \times \dfrac{1 \text{ h}}{\underset{3}{60 \text{ min}}} \times \dfrac{\overset{1}{20 \text{ drop}}}{\text{mL}} = 44 \text{ drops/min}$

   (c) 25% of 42 = .25 × 42 = 10.5 drop/min
   44 − 42 = 2 drop/min

   Since 2 drop/min is less than 10.5 drops/min, the adjustment is within the guidelines.

7. $\dfrac{750 \text{ mL}}{8 \text{ h}} \times \dfrac{1 \text{ h}}{\underset{4}{60 \text{ min}}} \times \dfrac{\overset{1}{15 \text{ drops}}}{\text{mL}} = 23 \text{ drops/min}$

8. $750 \text{ mL} \times \dfrac{h}{125 \text{ mL}} = 6 \text{ h}$ It will finish at 6 P.M. the same day.

9. $\dfrac{1000 \text{ mL}}{24 \text{ h}} = 42 \text{ mL/h}$ 10. $\dfrac{90 \text{ mL}}{h} \times \dfrac{1 \text{ h}}{\underset{3}{60 \text{ min}}} \times \dfrac{\overset{1}{20 \text{ drops}}}{\text{mL}} = 30 \text{ drops/min}$

11. $\dfrac{1000 \text{ mL}}{6 \text{ h}} = 167 \text{ mL/h}$ 12. $500 \text{ mL} \times \dfrac{h}{40 \text{ mL}} = 12.5 \text{ h}$ 13. $\dfrac{750 \text{ mL}}{24 \text{ h}} = 31 \text{ mL/h}$

14. $\dfrac{500 \text{ mL}}{3.25 \text{ h}} \times \dfrac{1 \text{ h}}{\underset{2}{60 \text{ min}}} \times \dfrac{\overset{1}{15 \text{ drops}}}{\text{mL}} = 38 \text{ drops/min}$

15. 32 mcdrop/min = 32 mL/h

   $6 \text{ h} \times \dfrac{32 \text{ mL}}{h} = 192 \text{ mL}$

Chapter 10

Diagnostic questions

1. Convert 60 mL per hour to mLs per minute. *Answer: 1 mL/min.*

2. Convert 25 mL per minute to L per hour. *Answer: 1.5 L/hr.*

3. A patient is to receive one dose of a drug at 5 mcg per kilogram body weight. He weighs 80 kg. How much of the drug should he have? *Answer: 400 mcg.*

4. Convert 40 mg per minute to mg per hour. *Answer: 2400 mg/h.*

5. A patient is receiving 900 mg of a drug over 90 minutes. How much of this drug would she have received after 1 hour? *Answer: 600 mg.*

Case study 10.1

1. $5{,}000 \text{ units} = ?\text{ mL} \quad \overset{1}{5{,}000} \text{ units} \times \dfrac{\text{mL}}{\underset{5}{25{,}000}} = \dfrac{1\text{ mL}}{5\text{ units}} = 0.2\text{ mL}$

$$18 \text{ unit/kg/hr} = 78 \text{ kg} \times \dfrac{18\text{ unit}}{\text{kg} \times \text{hr}}$$

$$= 1404 \text{ unit/hr}$$

Per day × 24 hr = 33,696 units/day

2. This rate is within the safe dosage range of 20 000–40 000 units per day.

3. Either 3 × 1 mg or 1 × 1 mg and 1 × 2 mg

4. 1000 mg/1 g × 5 mL/250 mg = 20 mL

5. ((150 mL × 3) + (330 mL × 2)) – 2000 mL = 890 mL

Try these for practice

1. 25 drops/min   2. 25 mL/h   3. 60 mg/h   4. 11 mcdrops/min   5. 12 mL/h

Exercises

1. $\dfrac{2\,\cancel{mcg}}{\text{min}} \times \dfrac{\cancel{mg}}{1000\,\cancel{mcg}} \times \dfrac{250\text{ mL}}{8\,\cancel{mg}} \times \dfrac{60\,\cancel{min}}{h} = 4\text{ mL/h}$

2. $\dfrac{\cancel{40}\text{ mL}}{\cancel{h}} \times \dfrac{1\,\cancel{h}}{\cancel{60}\text{ min}} \times \dfrac{1\,\cancel{g}}{\cancel{500}\text{ mL}} \times \dfrac{\overset{2}{\cancel{1000}}\text{ mg}}{1\,\cancel{g}} = 1.3\text{ mg/min}$

3. $91\,\cancel{kg} \times \dfrac{3\,\cancel{mcg}}{\cancel{kg}\cdot\cancel{min}} \times \dfrac{\cancel{60}\,\cancel{min}}{h} \times \dfrac{\cancel{mg}}{1000\,\cancel{mcg}} \times \dfrac{\cancel{250}\text{ mL}}{\cancel{400}\,\cancel{mg}} = 10\,\dfrac{\text{mL}}{h}$

4. $\dfrac{500\text{ mL}}{\underset{3}{\cancel{90}}\,\cancel{min}} \times \dfrac{\overset{2}{\cancel{60}}\,\cancel{min}}{h} = 333\,\dfrac{\text{mL}}{h}$ 5. $550\,\cancel{mL} \times \dfrac{h}{25\,\cancel{mL}} = 22\text{ h}$

6. $\dfrac{1000\,\cancel{units}}{h} \times \dfrac{1000\text{ mL}}{24\,000\,\cancel{units}} = 42\,\dfrac{\text{mL}}{h}$ 7. $\dfrac{1\,\cancel{mL}}{\cancel{min}} \times \dfrac{60\,\cancel{min}}{h} \times \dfrac{50\text{ units}}{500\,\cancel{mL}} = 6\text{ units/h}$

8. $\dfrac{40\,\cancel{mL}}{15\text{ min}} \times \dfrac{20\text{ drops}}{\cancel{mL}} = 53\text{ drops/min}$

9. $\dfrac{\text{drug}}{\text{weight} \times \text{time}} : \dfrac{20\,\cancel{mL}}{75\text{ kg}\,\cancel{h}} \times \dfrac{50\,\cancel{mg}}{250\,\cancel{mL}} \times \dfrac{1000\text{ mcg}}{1\,\cancel{mg}} \times \dfrac{1\,\cancel{h}}{60\text{ min}} = 0.89\text{ mcg/kg/min}$

10. (a) 4 mg (b) $4 \text{ mg} \times \dfrac{2 \text{ mL}}{5 \text{ mg}} = 1.6 \text{ mL}$ (c) 1.6 mL/min

11. $\dfrac{100 \text{ mL}}{60 \text{ min}} \times \dfrac{15 \text{ drops}}{\text{mL}} = 25 \text{ drops/min}$

12. $\dfrac{4 \text{ mcg}}{\text{min}} \times \dfrac{1 \text{ mg}}{1000 \text{ mcg}} \times \dfrac{500 \text{ mL}}{2 \text{ mg}} \times \dfrac{60 \text{ min}}{h} = 60 \text{ mL/h}$

13. $\dfrac{20 \text{ mL}}{h} \times \dfrac{500 \text{ mg}}{1000 \text{ mL}} = 10 \text{ mg/h}$

14. $82 \text{ kg} \times \dfrac{3 \text{ mcg}}{\text{kg} \cdot \text{min}} \times \dfrac{1 \text{ mg}}{1000 \text{ mcg}} \times \dfrac{250 \text{ mL}}{50 \text{ mg}} \times \dfrac{60 \text{ min}}{h} = 74 \text{ mL/h}$

15. $2.33 \text{ m}^2 \times \dfrac{75 \text{ mg}}{\text{m}^2} \times \dfrac{1 \text{ mL}}{50 \text{ mg}} = 3.5 \text{ mL}$

Chapter 11

Diagnostic questions

1. A child is to have a drug dose of 5 mg per kg body weight. This child is given 5 mg is this correct? *Answer: No – unless the child is 1 kg weight – the weight is needed to determine the final dose.*

2. Measure out 250 mg of an antibiotic. The dose in the bottle reads: 125 mg in 5 mLs. How many mLs do you give? *Answer: 10 mL.*

3. What is 40 mL multiplied by 20? *Answer: 800 mL or 0.8 L.*

4. What is 0.4 × 2.4 × 12? *Answer: 11.52.*

5. What is 0.75 × 0.30? *Answer: 0.225.*

Case study 11.1

1. $\left. \begin{array}{l} 10 \text{ kg} = \dfrac{40 \text{ mL}}{4} \\[4mm] 4 \text{ kg} = \dfrac{2 \text{ mL}}{\text{kg} \times h} = 8 \text{ mL} \end{array} \right\} \dfrac{48 \text{ mL}}{h} \times 24 = 1152 \text{ mL}$

2. 14 kg × 100 mg/kg/dy = 1400 mg/day (recommended)

   425 mg/dose × 4 doses/day = 1700 mg/day (prescribed)

   The prescribed dose is not safe – it is too high.

3. $\dfrac{50 \text{ mL}}{30 \text{ min}} \times \dfrac{60 \text{ min}}{h} = 100 \text{ mL/h}$

4. $14 \text{ kg} \times \dfrac{0.1 \text{ mg}}{\text{kg} \cdot \text{dose}} = 1.4 \text{ mg/dose (minimum)}$

   14 kg × 0.15 = 2.1 mg/dose (maximum dose)

   I mg is too low. Therefore, it is not a safe dose.

Try these for practice

1. $45 \text{ kg} \times \dfrac{0.1 \text{ unit}}{\text{kg}} = \dfrac{4.5 \text{ units}}{\text{dose}} \times \dfrac{2 \text{ doses}}{\text{day}} = 9 \text{ units per day}$

2. $0.62 \text{ m}^2 \times \dfrac{100 \text{ mg}}{\text{m}^2} = 62 \text{ mg (minimum)}$

   $0.62 \text{ m}^2 \times \dfrac{180 \text{ mg}}{\text{m}^2} = 111 \text{ mg (maximum)}$

   Since 90 is between 62 and 111, the dose is safe.

3. $250 \text{ mg} \times \dfrac{5 \text{ mL}}{125 \text{ mg}} = 10 \text{ mL}$ 4. $40 \text{ kg} \times \dfrac{0.3 \text{ mg}}{\text{kg}} \times \dfrac{5 \text{ mL}}{15 \text{ mg}} = 4 \text{ mL}$

5. $42 \text{ kg} = 60 \text{ mL/h} + 1 \text{ mL/kg/h over } 20 \text{ kg} = 22 \text{ ml}$

   $= 60 \text{ mL} + 22 \text{ mL} = 82 \text{ mL/h}$

   $= \text{maintenance } \dfrac{82 \text{ mL}}{\text{h}} \times 1.5$

   $= 123 \text{ mL/h (maintenance and a half)}$

Exercises

1. $18 \text{ kg} \times \dfrac{6 \text{ mg}}{\text{kg/day}} = 108 \text{ mg (minimum recommended)}$

   $18 \text{ kg} \times 7.5 \text{ mg/kg dose} = 135 \text{ mg (maximum recommended)}$

   Since 150 mg is higher than the maximum daily dose, the prescribed dose is not safe.

2. $4000 \text{ g} \times \dfrac{\text{kg}}{1000 \text{ g}} \times \dfrac{10 \text{ mg}}{\text{kg}} = 40 \text{ mg}$

3. $\text{BSA} = \sqrt{\dfrac{106 \times 23}{3600}} = \sqrt{0.677} = 0.82 \text{ m}^2$

   $0.82 \text{ m}^2 \times 7.5 \text{ mg/m}^2 = 6.15 \text{ mg (minimum)}$

   $0.82 \text{ m}^2 \times 30 \text{ mg/m}^2 = 24.6 \text{ mg (maximum)}$

   Since the prescribed dose of 2.9 mg is below the recommended minimum dose, it is not safe.

4. $32 \text{ kg} \times \dfrac{10 \text{ mg}}{\text{kg}} = 320 \text{ mg}$

5. $1.2 \text{ m}^2 \times \dfrac{350 \text{ mg}}{\text{m}^2 \cdot \text{day}} = 420 \text{ mg/day (minimum)}$

   $1.2 \text{ m}^2 \times \dfrac{450 \text{ mg}}{\text{m}^2 \cdot \text{day}} = 540 \text{ mg/day (maximum)}$

   The safe dose range for the child is 420–540 mg/day.

6. $35 \text{ kg} \times \dfrac{30 \text{ mg}}{\text{kg/day}} \times \dfrac{\text{mL}}{185} = 5.6 \text{ mL/day}$

$\dfrac{5.6 \text{ mL}}{\cancel{\text{day}}} \times \dfrac{\cancel{\text{day}}}{3 \text{ doses}} = 1.8 \text{ mL per dose}$

7. $\dfrac{65 \text{ mL}}{\text{h}} = 65 \text{ mcdrop/min}$

8. $23 \text{ kg} \times \dfrac{2 \text{ mg}}{\text{kg/day}} = 46 \text{ mg/day (minimum dose)}$

$23 \text{ kg} \times \dfrac{4 \text{ mg}}{\text{kg/day}} = 92 \text{ mg /day (maximum dose)}$

Since 90 mg/day (30 mg × 3) is between 46 mg and 92 mg it is safe and since one dose of 30 mg is less than 50 mg the prescribed dose is safe.

9. (a) $25 \text{ kg} = 60 \text{ mL/h} + 1 \text{ mL/kg/h}$

$= 60 \text{ mL/h} + 5 \text{ mL/h}$

$= 65 \text{ mL/h} \times 24 \text{ h}$

$= 1560 \text{ mL/day (maintenance)}$

(b) 65 mL/h

10. $0.82 \text{ } \cancel{\text{m}^2} \times \dfrac{2\,000\,000 \text{ units}}{\cancel{\text{m}^2}} = 1\,640\,000 \text{ units}$

11. $1.2 \text{ } \cancel{\text{g}} \times \dfrac{1000 \text{ } \cancel{\text{mg}}}{1 \text{ } \cancel{\text{g}}} \times \dfrac{\text{mL}}{60 \text{ } \cancel{\text{mg}}} = 20 \text{ mL}$

12. $1.1 \text{ } \cancel{\text{m}^2} \times \dfrac{160 \text{ } \cancel{\text{mg}}}{\cancel{\text{m}^2}} \times \dfrac{10 \text{ mL}}{100 \text{ } \cancel{\text{mg}}} = 17.6 \text{ mL}$

13. $14.5 \text{ } \cancel{\text{kg}} \times \dfrac{30 \text{ mg}}{\cancel{\text{kg}} \cdot \text{day}} = 435 \text{ mg/day (minimum)}$ ⎫
⎬ recommended
$14.5 \text{ } \cancel{\text{kg}} \times \dfrac{50 \text{ mg}}{\cancel{\text{kg}} \cdot \text{day}} = 725 \text{ mg/day (maximum)}$ ⎭

(a) Safe Range = 435 – 725 mg, this dose is 125 mg × 6 = 750 mg; it is over the upper safe limit and thus not safe.

(b) Seek advice from prescriber (dose too high)

14. $41 \text{ kg} \times 40 \text{ mg/kg/day} = 1640 \text{ mg/day}$

$1640\text{/day} \times \text{day/4 doses} = 410 \text{ mg/dose}$

$410 \text{ mg} \times \dfrac{\text{mL}}{50 \text{ mg}} = 8.2 \text{ mL}$

Thus 200 mL sodium chloride plus 8.2 mg Vancomycin = 208.2 mL

208.2 mL/90 min × 60 min/h = 138 mL/h

15. $\dfrac{100 \text{ mg}}{20 \text{ min}} = 5 \text{ mg/min}$

278

Cumulative review exercises

Chapters 1–4

1. 125 micrograms   2. 9 mg   3. 5650 g   4. 100 micrograms   5. 60 mg
6. 7.65 g   7. 7750 mL   8. 600 mcg   9. 1.25 L   10. 0.01 g   11. 0.09 g

Chapters 5–8

12. 10.8 mL   13. 3 tab   14. 4 tab   15. 3 tab   16. 3 tab   17. 60 mL
18. 50 mL of H_2O and 150 mL of Isocal   19. 0.6 mg   20. 0.0004 g   21. 250 mcg
22. 0.2 mg   23. quinapril HCl   24. PO   25. store below 25°c   26. 8 tab
27. 2 tab   28. Cipramil   29. 40 mg/mL   30. 0.5 mL   31. 30 doses

Chapters 9–11

32. 4.5 mg   33. 40 mL/h   34. 156 mL/h   35. 17 drops/min   36. 2.11 m^2
37. 1 capsule   38. 80 mL/h   39. 3 mL   40. 1.7 mL   41. 10 mL   42. 10 mL
43. 525 mg   44. 30 units   45. (a) 200 mg (b) 1 tab   46. 50 units   47. 20 mL
48. (a) 2 cap (b) 0.3 g   49. 60 drops/min   50. 11:42 A.M. the next day (14 h 42 min)

Comprehensive self-tests

Comprehensive self-test 1

1. 735 mg   2. 0.1 g   3. 8 h 20 min   4. 12.5 g   5. 2 tab   6. (a) 100 mL/h (b) 1000 mg
7. 0.33 mL

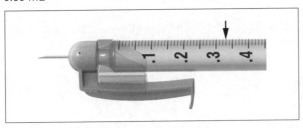

8. 3 mL/h   9. 6.8 units/h   10. 2.5 mL   11. (a) 0.22 mg/d (b) 0.32 mg/d (c) yes
12. (a) 158 mg (b) 197 mL   13. 25 drops/min   14. 0.5 mL
15. (a) 1.3 mL/min (b) 25 drops/min (c) 13 h 20 min   16. 2040 mL
17. 30 mL (1 dose) 120 mL (1 day)   18. (a) 10 mg (b) 60 mL
19. (a) 0.009 mg (b) 21 mL/h

Comprehensive self-test 2

1. 2000 units   2. (a) 19.2 mg (b) 3.8 mL   3. 2 tab   4. 2.2 mL
5. (a) yes (b) 1.1 mL   6. 0900h the next day   7. 12.5 mL

8. (a) 2 mL

(b)

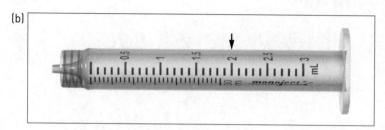

9. (a) 216 mg/d (b) 675 mg/d   10. 2.25 g   11. 100 mL/h   12. 432 mL daily 18 mL/h
13. yes   14. 120 mL/h   15. 2.5 mL   16. 30 mL   17. 21 mL/h
18. 0.7 mL   19. (a) 1 mL (b) 3 mL or 2 mL   20. 0400 h the next day.

Comprehensive self-test 3

1. 1260 mL   2. 8 mL   3. 1.2 mL   4. 1600 units/h and it is safe.
5. 16 200 mg   6. 0.35 mL   7. No (76 mg)   8. 30 mL   9. 27 mL/h and 653 mL

10.

Insulatard   Actrapid

11. BSA 1.63, 32 600 units   12. 42 mL/h   13. 0505 h the next day   14. 3 tab
15. 0.3 g   16. 75 drops/min   17. 2 tab   18. 0.51 m^2 19. 1128 mL

Comprehensive self-test 4

1. yes (safe range is 70.4–87.9 mg)   2. 2.7 mL   3. 2 tab   4. 8 h   5. 240 mL
6. 0.4 mL   7. 0.2 mL   8. 2 mL/min   9. 5 mL/min   10. 32.4 mg
11. 1047 mL (26 lb = 11.81 kg)   12. Yes (range 180–360 mg)   13. 20 units/h
14. 0.5 mL   15. Yes (daily 2000 mg same as 500 mg 6 hrly)

Reference

Nursing and Midwifery Council (NMC) (2007) *Standards for Medicines Managements*. London: Nursing and Midwifery Council. Available at http://www.nmcuk.org/aDisplayDocument.aspx?DocumentID= 3251 accessed March 2009.

Appendix B
Common abbreviations used in medical documentation

To someone unfamiliar with prescriptive abbreviations, medication orders may look like a foreign language. To interpret a prescription accurately and to administer drugs safely, a qualified person must have a thorough knowledge of common abbreviations. For instance, when the prescriber writes, 'Morphine sulphate (Oromorph) 15 mg PO 4 hourly prn' the administrator knows how to interpret it as 'Morphine sulphate, 15 milligrams, by mouth, every four hours, whenever necessary.' For measurement abbreviations, refer to Appendix C.

Abbreviation	Meaning
ac	before meals *(ante cibum)*
A.M., am	morning
b.i.d. or bd	two times a day
BP	blood pressure
C	Celsius; centigrade
cap	capsule
CVP	central venous pressure
FBC	full blood count
g	gram
h, hr	hour
ID	intradermal
IM	intramuscular
IV	intravenous
kg	kilogram
L	litre
MAR	medication administration record
mcg	microgram
mcdrop, μdrop	microdrop
mg	milligram
min	minute
mL	millilitre
mmol	millimole
n, nocte	night
NGT	nasogastric tube
NKA	no known allergies
NaCl	normal saline

Abbreviation	Meaning
NSAID	nonsteroidal anti-inflammatory drug
OTC	over the counter
P	pulse
PEG	percutaneous endoscopic gastrostomy tube
PEJ	percutaneous endoscopic jejunostomy
PICC	peripherally inserted central catheter
P.M., pm	afternoon, evening
PO	by mouth *(per os)*
post-op	after surgery
PR	by way of the rectum
pre-op	before surgery
prn	when required or whenever necessary
q.i.d. or qds	four times a day *(quarter in die)*
R e.g. TPR	respiration
SL	sublingual
SR	sustained release
stat	immediately *(statum)*
subcut	subcutaneous
supp	suppository
T	temperature
t.i.d. or tds	three times a day *(ter in die)*
TPN	total parenteral nutrition

Appendix C
Tables of weight conversions

Use the following tables to convert between the metric kilogram and imperial measurements

Table C.1 Pounds and stones to to kilograms

lb	stones	kg	lb	stones	kg	lb	stones	kg
2.2		1.0	120		54.5	238	17 stones	108.2109.1
5		2.3	126	9 stones	57.27	245		111.4
10		4.5	130		59.1	252	18 stones	114.5
14	1 stone	6.36.8	135		61.4	255		115.9
20		9.1	140	10 stones	63.6	260		118.2
28	2 stones	12.72	145		65.9	266	19 stones	120.9
30		13.6	150		68.2	270		122.7
35		15.9	154	11 stones	70	275		125
42	3 stones	19	160		72.7	280	20 stones	127.3
45		20.5	165		75	285		129.5
50		22.7	168	12 stones	76.36	290		131.8
56	4 stones	25.4	175		79.5	294	21 stones	133.63
60		27.3	180		81.8	300		136.4
65		29.5	182	13 stones	82.72	305		138.6
70	5 stones	31.8	190		86.4	308	22 stones	140.
75		34.1	196	14 stones	89	315		143.2
80		36.4	200		90.9	322	23 stones	146.36
84	6 stones	38.18	205		93.2	325		147.7
90		40.9	210	15 stones	95.5	330		150
95		43.2	215		97.7	336	24 stones	152.72
98	7 stones	44.5	220		100	340		154.5
105		47.7	224	16 stones	101.8	345		156.8
112	8 stones	50.9	230		104.5	350	25 stones	159.1
115		52.3	235		106.8	355		161.4

Table C.2 Kilograms to pounds and stones

kg	lb	stones	kg	lb	stones	kg	lb	stones
2	4.4		56	123.2		110	242	
4	8.8		57.27	126	9 stones	112	246.4	
6.36	14	1 stone	60	132		114.5	252	18 stones
8	17.6		62	136.4		116	255.2	
10	22		63.6	140.	10 stones	118	259.6	
12.72	28	2 stones	66	145.2		120.9	266	19 stones
14	30.8		68	149.6		122	268.4	
16	35.2		70	154	11 stones	124	272.8	
18	39.6		72	158.4		126	277.2	
19	42	3 stones	74	162.8		127.2	280	20 stones
22	48.4		76.36	168	12 stones	130	286	
24	52.8		78	171.6		132	290.4	
25.46	56	4 stones	80	176		133.6	294	21 stones
28	61.6		82.7	182	13 stones	136	299.2	
30	66		84	184.8		138	303.6	
31.8	70.	5 stones	86	189.2		140	308	22 stones
34	74.8		88	193.6		142	312.4	
36	79.2		89	196	14 stones	144	316.8	
38.18	84	6 stones	92	202.4		146.3	322	23 stones
40	88		94	206.8		148	325.6	
42	92.4		95.4	210	15 stones	150	330	
44.5	98	7 stones	98	215.6		152.7	336	24 stones
46	101.2		100	220		154	338.8	
48	105.6		101.8	224	16 stones	156	343.2	
50.9	112	8 stones	104	228.8		158	347.6	
52	114.4		106	233.2		159	350	25 stones
54	118.8		108.18	238	17 stones	162	356.4	

Appendix D
Ratio and algebraic calculations

There are a number of methods which can be used to calculate drug doses and rates. Here is a summary of the most poplar though not always the most well understood – use these when you are confident and proficient in the methods outlined in earlier chapters.

Formulas include:

$$\text{Amount to administer} = \frac{\text{Desired dose}}{\text{Dose on hand}} \times \text{Quantity on hand}$$

Another technique uses a ratio and proportion approach (using algebra principles), which is useful only in the simplest problems, and is illustrated in the following examples.

Example D.1

If each tablet contains 5 mg, how many tablets contain 15 mg?

The information in the example is summarised in the following table:

Known equivalent	1 tablet = 5 mg
Unknown equivalent	x tables = 15 mg

The equivalents in the table are written as fractions (ratios) and are equated to form the following proportion:

$$\frac{1 \text{ tab}}{5 \text{ mg}} = \frac{x \text{ tab}}{15 \text{ mg}}$$

x is found by algebraically solving the proportion:

$$\frac{1}{5} = \frac{x}{15}$$

Now, cross-multiply:

$$\frac{1}{5} \bcancel{\times} \frac{x}{15}$$

$$5x = 15$$

Now, divide both sides by 5:

$$\frac{5x}{5} = \frac{15}{5}$$

Cancel:

$$\frac{5x}{5} = \frac{\overset{3}{\cancel{15}}}{\cancel{5}}$$

$$x = 3$$

So, 3 tablets contain 15 mg.

Example D.2

A vial label states: $\dfrac{75 \text{ mg}}{5 \text{ mL}}$. How many millilitres of this solution contains 10 milligrams

of the drug?

The information in the example is summarised in the following table:

Known equivalent	75 mg = 5 mL
Unknown equivalent	10 mg = x mL

The equivalents in the table are written as fractions (ratios) and are equated to form the following proportion:

$$\frac{75 \text{ mg}}{5 \text{ mL}} = \frac{10 \text{ mg}}{x \text{ mL}}$$

x is found by algebraically solving the proportion:

$$\frac{75}{5} = \frac{10}{x}$$

Now, cross-multiply:

$$\frac{75}{5} \diagdown \frac{10}{x}$$

$$50 = 75x$$

Now, divide both sides by 75:

$$\frac{50}{75} = \frac{75x}{75}$$

Cancel:

$$\frac{\overset{2}{\cancel{50}}}{\underset{3}{\cancel{75}}} = \frac{\cancel{75}x}{\cancel{75}}$$

$$x = \frac{2}{3} \quad \text{or} \quad 0.67$$

So, 0.67 mL contains 10 mg of the drug.

Example D.3

If an IV containing 880 mL is to infuse in 8 hours, then how long will it take for 350 mL of this IV to infuse?

The information in the example is summarised in the following table:

Known equivalent	880 mL = 8 h
Unknown equivalent	350 mL = x h

The equivalents in the table are written as fractions (ratios) and are equated to form the proportion below:

$$\frac{880 \text{ mL}}{8 \text{ h}} = \frac{350 \text{ mL}}{x \text{ h}}$$

x is found by algebraically solving the proportion:

$$\frac{880}{8} = \frac{350}{x}$$

Now, cross-multiply:

$$\frac{880}{8} \diagdown \frac{350}{x}$$

$$880x = 2800$$

Now, divide both sides by 880:

$$\frac{880x}{880} = \frac{2800}{880}$$

Cancel:

$$\frac{880x}{880} = \frac{2800}{880}$$

$$x = \frac{2800}{880} \quad \text{or} \quad 3.18$$

So, it will take about 3.18 hours for 350 mL to infuse.

To change 0.18 h to minutes, ratio and proportion could also be used.

Known equivalent	1 h = 60 min
Unknown equivalent	0.18 h = x min

The equivalents in the table are written as fractions (ratios) and are equated to form the proportion below:

$$\frac{1 \text{ h}}{60 \text{ min}} = \frac{0.18 \text{ h}}{x \text{ min}}$$

x is found by algebraically solving the proportion:

$$\frac{1}{60} = \frac{0.18}{x}$$

Now, cross-multiply:

$$\frac{1}{60} \diagdown \frac{0.18}{x}$$

$$10.8 = x$$

So, it will take about 3 hours and 11 minutes for 350 mL to infuse.

Index